CURRENT TRENDS IN TRANSPLANTATION

DRUG THERAPY AND MONITORING

Gary A. Levy, MD
University Health Network – University of Toronto
Toronto, Canada

John R. Lake, MD
University of Minnesota Medical Center
Fairview, Minnesota USA

David W. Holt, DSc (Med), FRCPath
St. George's, University of London, UK

Pierre Wallemacq, PhD, EurClin Chem
Cliniques Universitaires St Luc
Brussels, Belgium

Abbott Laboratories / Abbott Park

CURRENT TRENDS IN TRANSPLANTATION: DRUG THERAPY AND MONITORING

ISBN 978-0-692-00418-0

TABLE OF CONTENTS

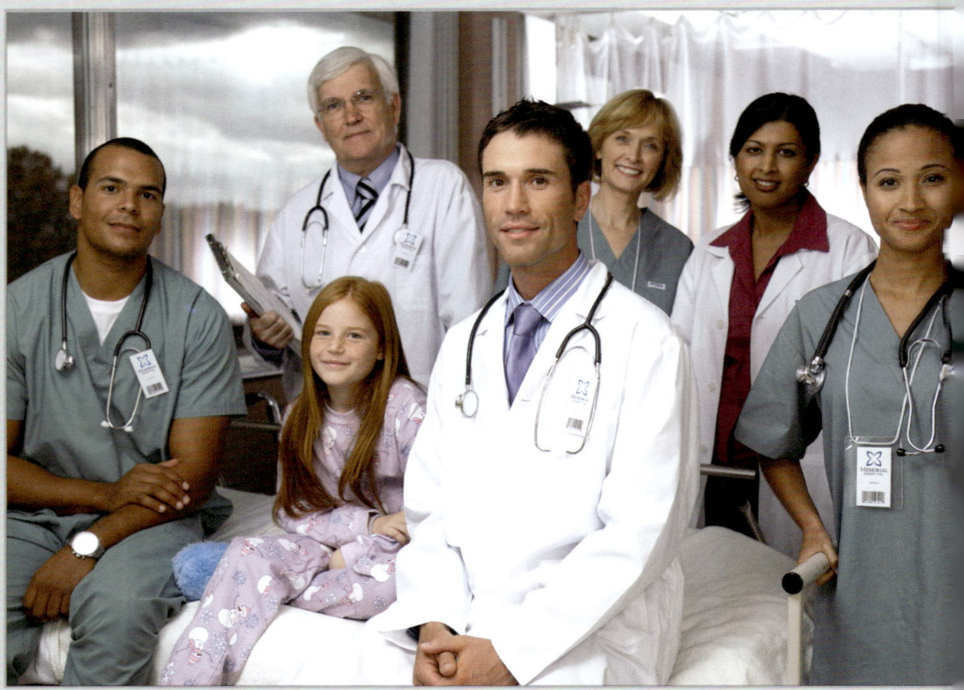

OVERVIEW

Solid organ transplantation has now become a highly effective therapy for patients with end-stage organ failure. This is largely due to advances in surgical techniques as well as to the introduction of highly effective immunosuppressive agents which can be monitored using reproducible and sensitive laboratory assay systems.

Thus, approximately 50,000 solid organ transplants are performed each year with 1 and 5 year survival rates approximating 80-90%.

Despite these tremendous achievements, long-term survival is limited by toxicity of immunosuppressive agents and sub-clinical and chronic rejection.

Advances in our understanding of immunology of transplantation has now generated newer classes of immunosuppressive agents which have the potential to improve long-term outcomes further and to lessen the need for the established agents, including the calcineurin inhibitors, cyclosporine and tacrolimus.

For this to occur, a coordinated and integrated approach to care involving surgeons, physicians, nurses and laboratory personnel must be employed.

This monograph discusses the advances in our understanding of the immunology of transplantation, the present state of immunosuppressive drug therapy, newer advances in diagnosis and treatment of rejection and monitoring strategies to maximize use of immunosuppressive agents. In addition, genomic and proteomic approaches to induce tolerance and the ability to maintain long-term graft survival without the need for immunosuppression are considered.

Gary Levy, MD

Toronto, Canada

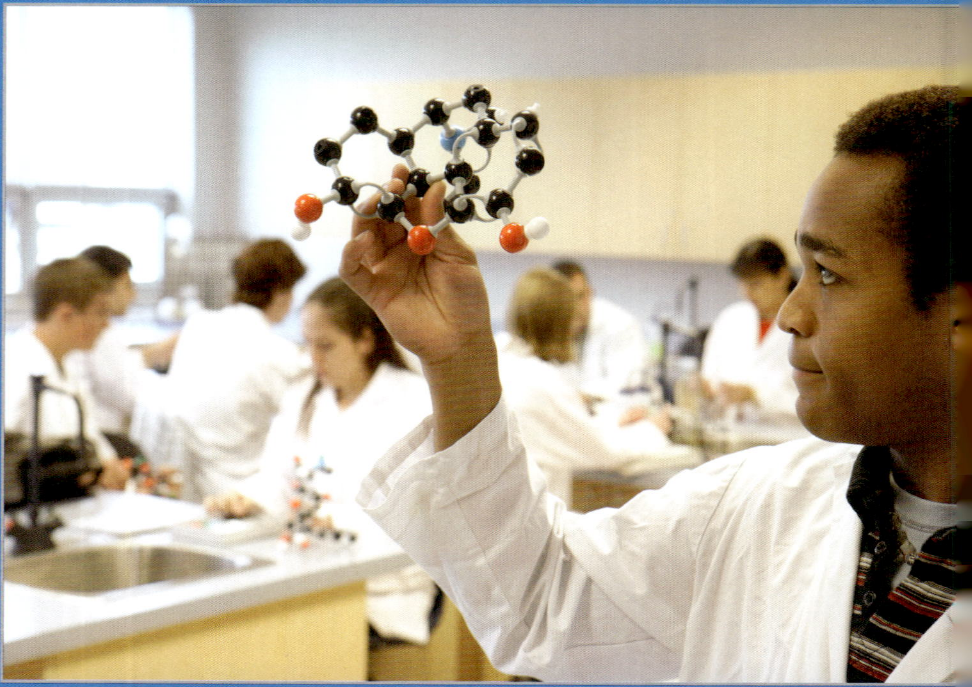

CHAPTER 1 CONTENTS

HISTORY OF SOLID ORGAN TRANSPLANTATION

Currently, transplantation of tissues and organs is the only truly effective therapy for patients with end stage organ failure. The growth of visceral surgery at the end of the 19th century allowed for successful removal of donor organs. The success of Carrel in 1901 to perform vascular anastomoses allowed experiments to proceed in which removed organs could be implanted successfully into animals. Through the early 20th century, a number of laboratories implanted kidneys into animals, setting the stage for human renal transplantation to proceed.

In 1906, Jaboulay was the first to attempt renal transplantation in a human. In two cases, he used organs from animals and, although the surgery was successful, both grafts were rejected by a process today termed xenotransplant rejection. Following other unsuccessful attempts in the USA and Russia, even in some cases using human organs, in 1953 Murray and Hume successfully transplanted cadaveric kidneys from humans, resulting in 5 month patient and graft survival. In 1954 the first successful human transplant between two identical twins was performed by a team headed by Murray, at the Brigham Hospital in Boston. Dr. Murray later shared the Nobel Prize for Medicine for his efforts in organ and cell transplantation.

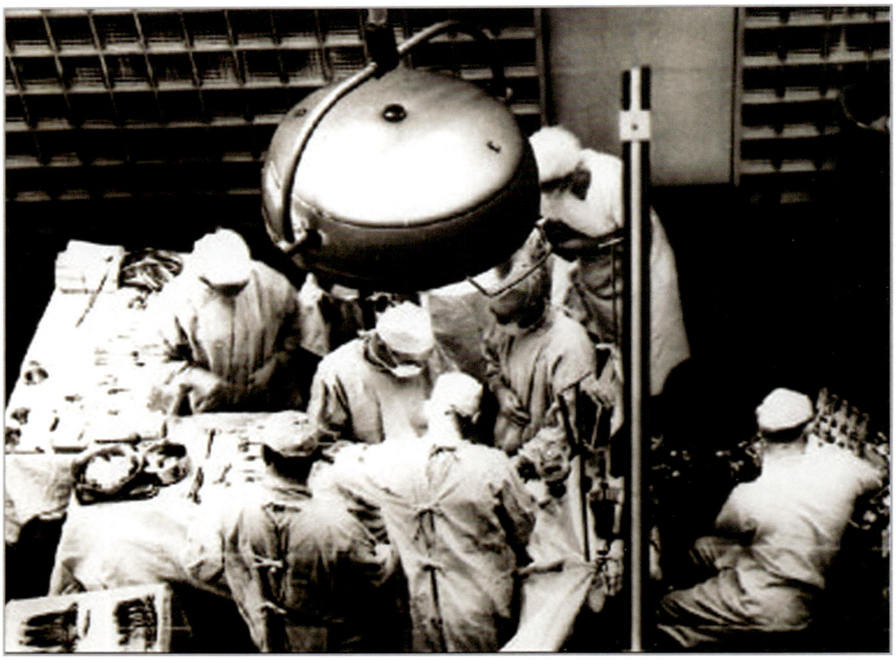

FIGURE 1-1. Dr. Murray's surgical team performing the first successful kidney transplant.

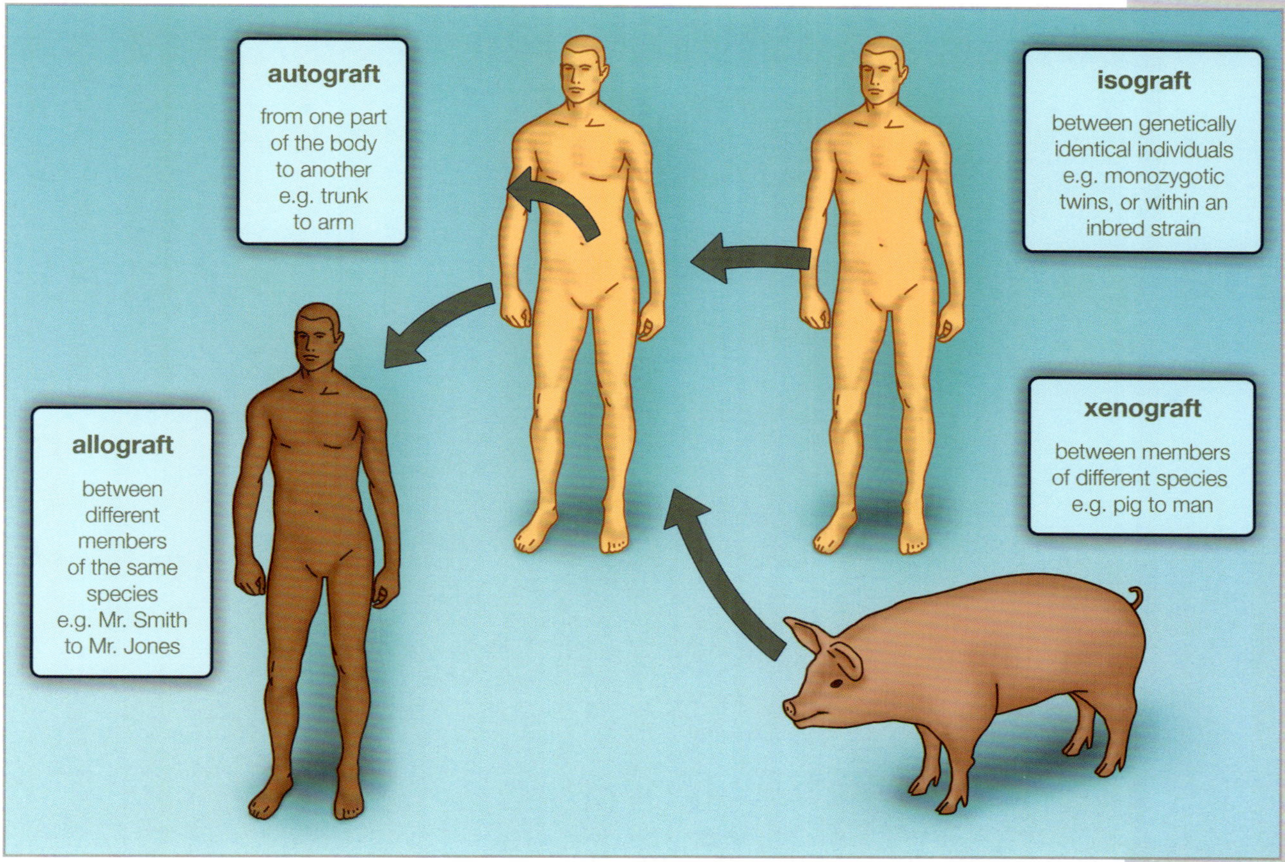

FIGURE 1-2. Genetic barriers to transplantation.

With the advent of effective immunosuppressive agents, including azathioprine and, in 1980 cyclosporine, it became possible to perform allogeneic renal transplants and heart, liver and lung transplantation became possible.

TABLE 1-1. History of Transplantation

Date	Event	Surgeon	Location
1902	First experimental kidney transplant	Emerich Ullmann	Vienna
1906	Sheep and pig kidneys transplanted into two humans	Mathieu Jaboulay	Lyon, France
	Technique for vascular anastamosis	Alexis Carrel	France
	Corneal transplant	Eduard Zirm	Austria
1914	Technical problems solved but transplant would not succeed until tolerance was achieved	Alexis Carrel	France
1930's	6 cadaveric renal transplants	Yu Yu Voronoy	Russia
1950's	Renal transplants from convict donors		France
	Mother to son kidney transplant	Jean Hamburger	France
	9 cadaveric renal transplants	David Hume	Boston, USA
1954	Kidney transplanted from one identical twin brother to the other – kidney functioned immediately	John Merrill, J. Hartwell Harrison & Joseph Murray	Boston, USA
1962	1st successful cadaveric kidney transplant	David Hume	Boston, USA
1963	1st liver transplant	Thomas Starzl	Denver, USA
1963	1st lung transplant	Hardy	USA
1966	1st pancreas transplant	W.D. Kelly et al	Minnesota, USA
1967	1st heart transplant	Christiaan Barnard	South Africa
1978	1st islet transplant	Paul Lacey	St. Louis, USA
1981	1st heart-lung transplant	Bruce Reitz	Stanford University
1983	1st lung lobe transplant	Joel Cooper	Toronto, CAN
1991	1st successful small intestine transplant	Revillon	Paris, France
1998	1st hand transplant	Earl Owen	Australia
2005	1st face transplant	Jean-Michel Dubernard	France
2008	1st trachea transplant from stem cells	Paolo Machiarini	Barcelona

PIONEERS IN TRANSPLANTATION

Today, worldwide, approximately 50,000 solid organ transplants are performed each year, of which 60% are kidneys. Despite active programs to encourage organ donation, the gap between supply and demand continues to widen and many patients do not get access to life saving organ transplantation. However, despite the improved success of short and long-term results for transplantation, the shortage of human donor organs, the need for long-term immunosuppression, and the loss of organs to chronic allograft injury limits the success of this therapy.

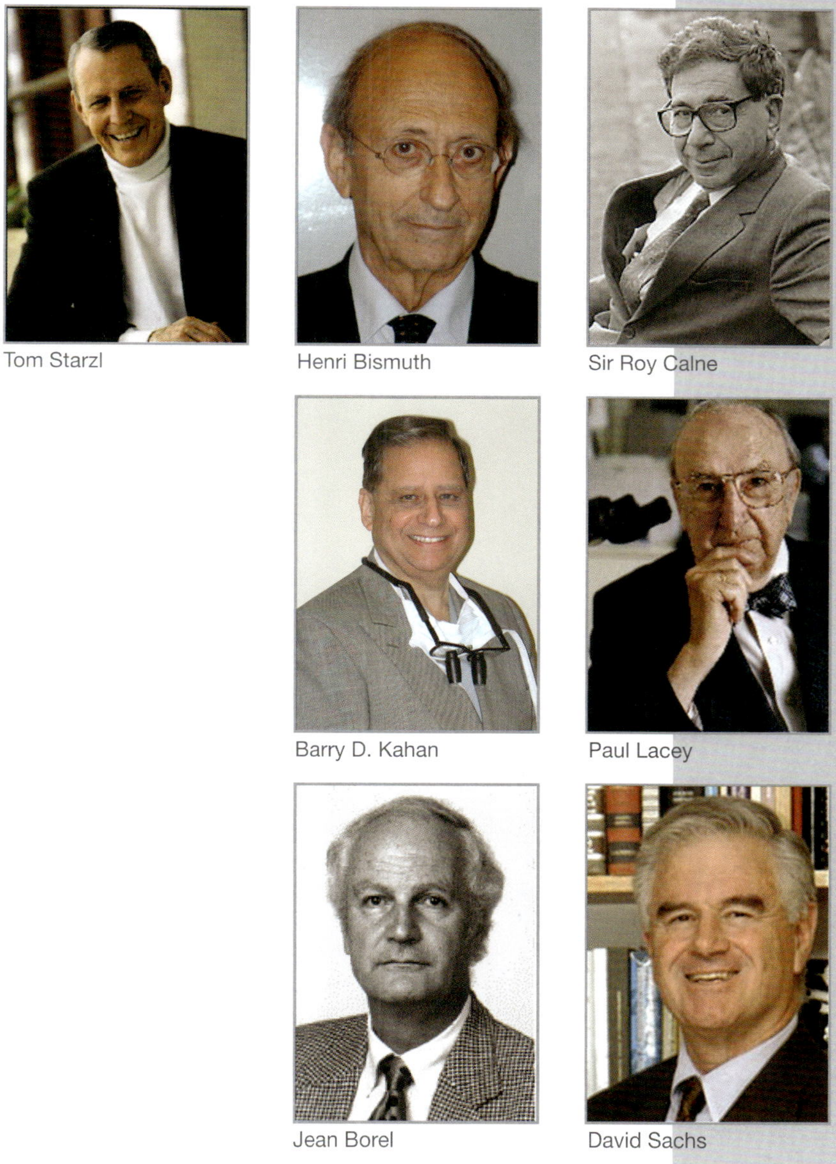

FIGURE 1-3. Key researchers and clinicians who pioneered the field of solid organ transplantation. Pictures courtesy of T. Starzl, R. Calne, B. Kahan, D. Sachs, H. Bismuth, and Am J. Transplant. (P. Lacey).

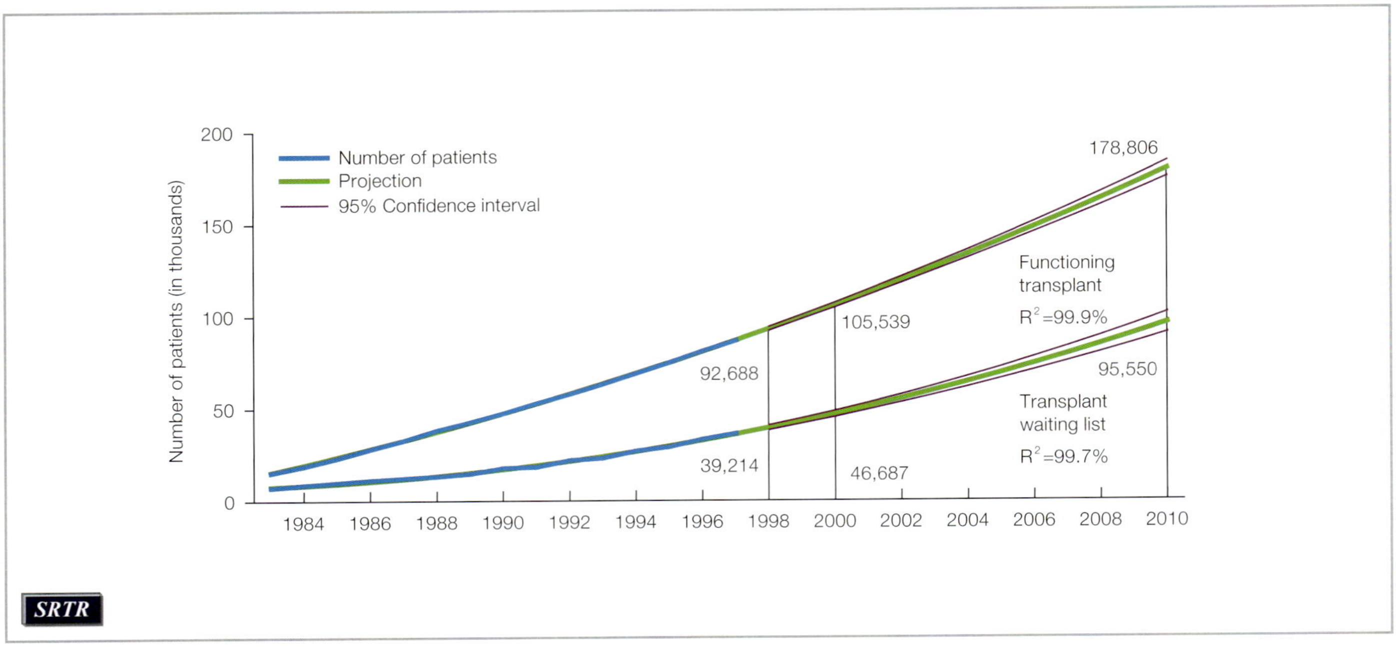

FIGURE 1-4. Demand for solid organ transplantation. Data from UNOS SRTR database.

Even though the number of patients with a functioning graft has increased over the past twenty years so has the number of patients on the transplant waiting list. This is due to the increased demand for solid organ transplantation relative to the supply of donor organs.

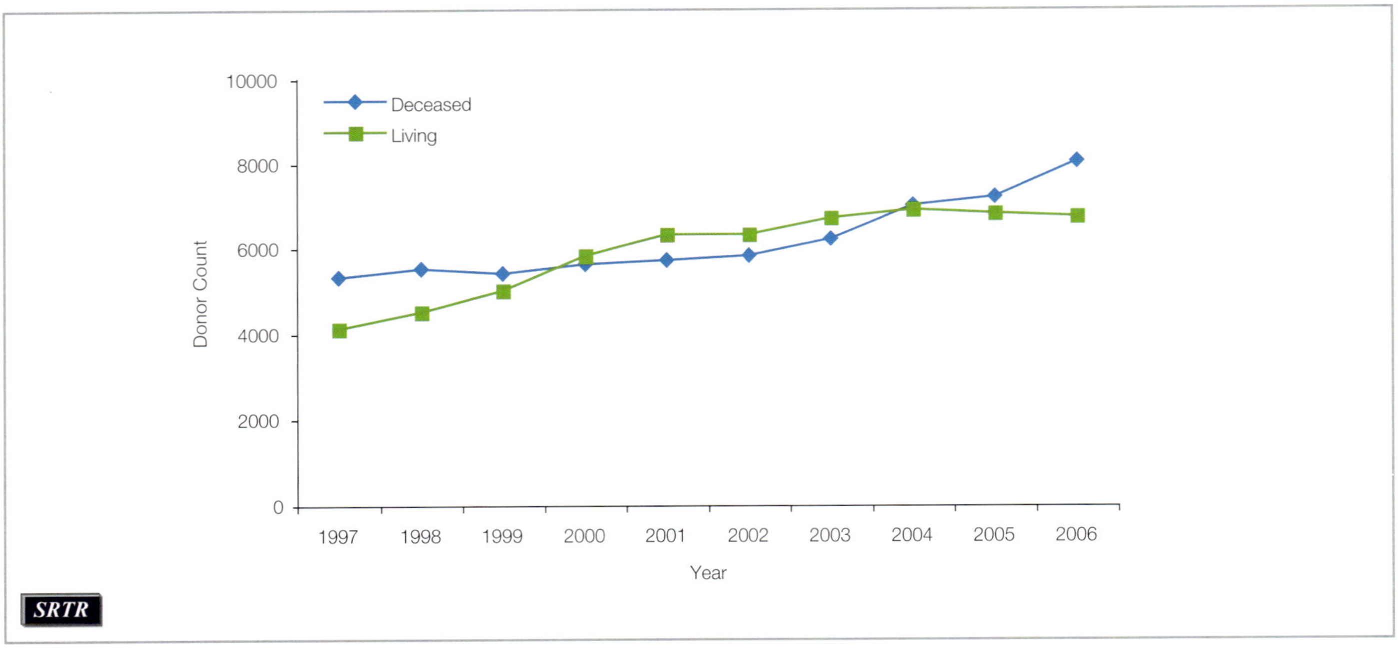

FIGURE 1-5. Total number of deceased and living donors of all organs recovered for transplant. Data from 2007 OPTN/SRTR Annual Report, 1997-2006. HHS/HRSA/HSB/DOT. Table 1.1.

There has been a modest increase in both deceased and living organ donors over the past 10 years.

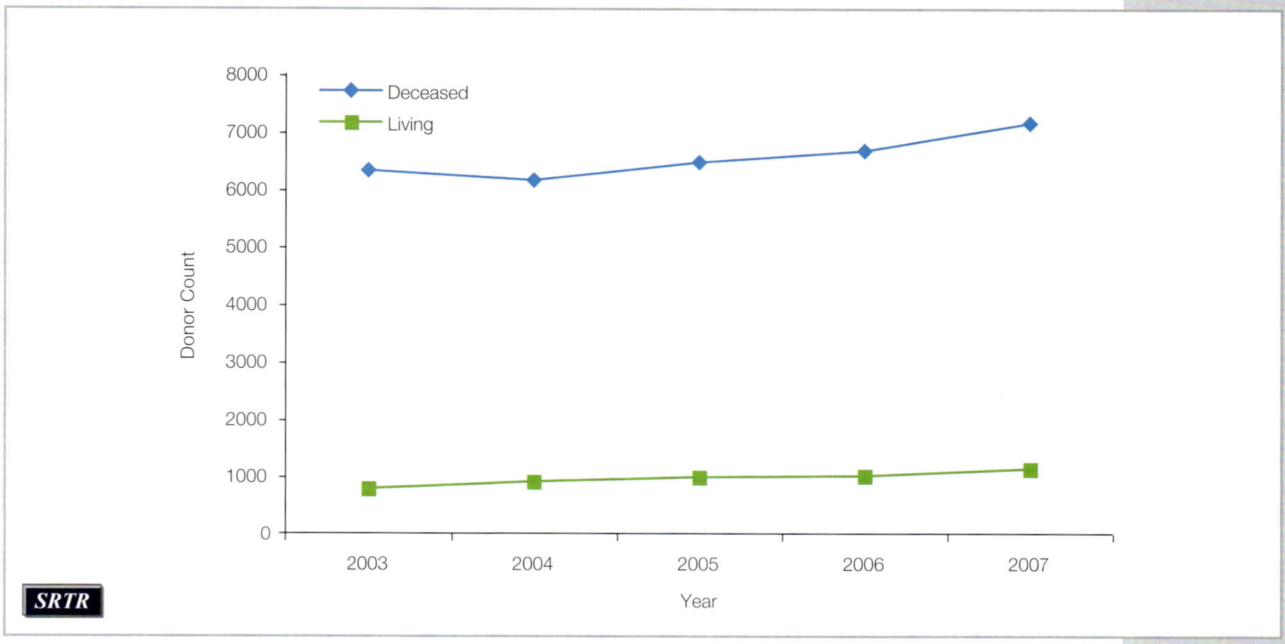

FIGURE 1-6. Number of transplanted organs by donor type. Data from Eurotransplant Annual Report 2007, Table 2.7.

To increase the number of available organs, the transplant community has now created expanded criteria for donation (ECD) as shown in Figure 1-7. In some areas, the number of ECD kidneys available for transplantation exceed the number of standard criteria for donation (SCD) kidneys.

TABLE 1-2. Standard Criteria for Donation (SCD)

	Liver	Lung	Heart	Kidney
Age	<55	30-40	<55	<55
Risk Factors	-Negative HCV -Negative HIV -Negative HBV -Steatosis <10% -NHBD <75 min. asystole	-Ischemia time 4 hrs. -$pO_2 \geq 25$ mm Hg -Normal CXR	-Normal coronary arteries -Normal CO	-serum creatinine <1.8 mg/dL (159.1 µmol/L) -NHBD -No hypertension -No atherosclerosis

HCV, Hepatitis C virus; HIV, Human Immunodeficiency virus; HBV, Hepatitis B virus; Steatosis, abnormal lipid retention; NHBD, Non-Heart Beating Donor; asystole, no cardiac activity; Ischemia, shortage of blood supply to an organ; CXR, Chest X-Ray; CO, Cardiac Output.

TABLE 1-3. Extended Criteria for Donation (ECD)

	Liver	Lung	Heart	Kidney
Age	N/A	70	55	70
Serum Creatinine	-	-	-	2.0 mg/dL (176.2 µmol/L)
Shock/Cardiac Arrest	75 min.	-	-	90 min.
Hypertension	-	-	-	-
Atherosclerosis	Mild	Mild	Mild	Mild
Glomerulosclerosis	-	-	-	<20%
Coronary Angiograms	-	-	Near normal	-
CXR	-	Near normal	Normal	-
Steatosis	30-40%	-	-	-

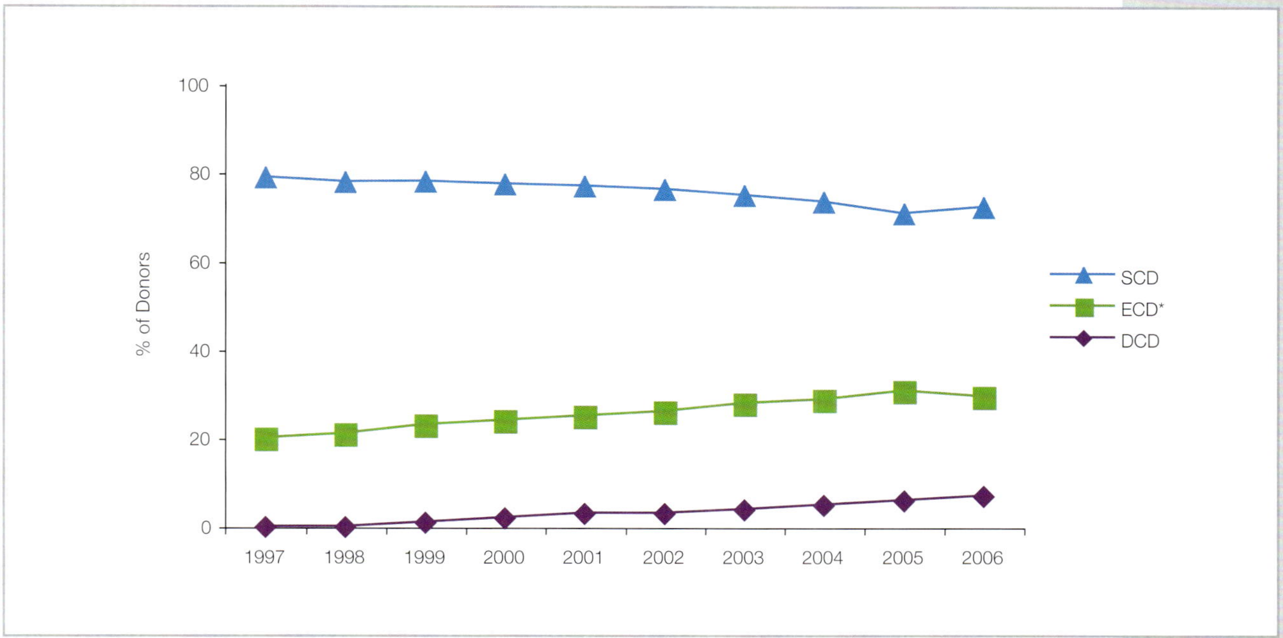

*Includes donation after cardiac death (DCD) that meet ECD criteria

FIGURE 1-7. Deceased donor population, by donor type and year (percentage). Data from 2007 OPTN/SRTR Annual Report, 1997-2006. HHS/HRSA/HSB/DOT. Table 2.12.

However, despite the improved success of short and long-term results of transplantation, there continues to be loss of organs to chronic allograft injury which limits the success of transplantation. Figure 1-8 shows the causes of renal graft loss after the first year. Chronic Allograft Nephropathy (CAN), also now called interstitial fibrosis with tubular atrophy, is the leading cause of graft loss. CAN is a term used to describe progressive tissue damage leading to allograft dysfunction. In Figure 1-9 a comparison of projected half-lives versus actual Kaplan-Meier half-lives in deceased donor transplants indicates a modest 2 year increase in actual half-lives, significantly less than the projected half-lives.

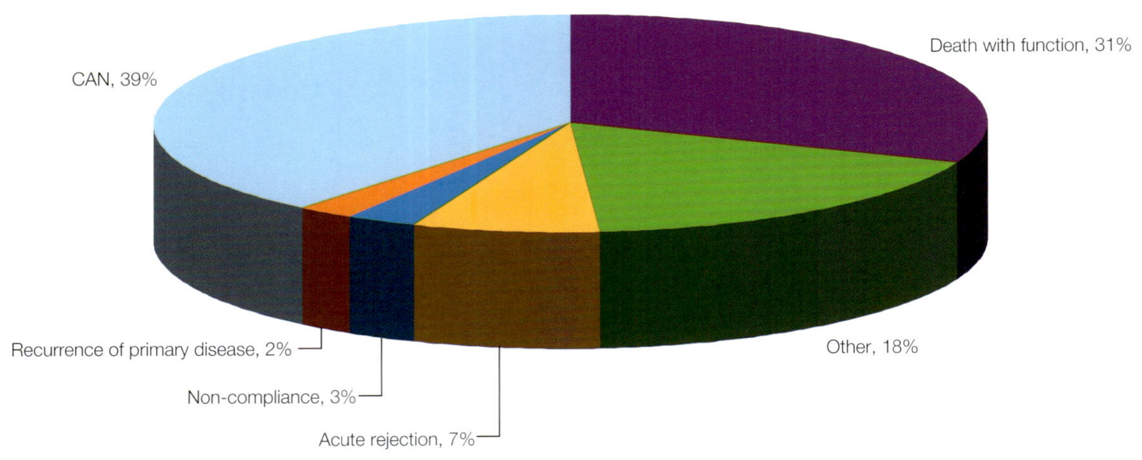

FIGURE 1-8. Causes of renal graft loss after first year (120,000 transplants, 15,000 failures). Data from UNOS 1987-2001.

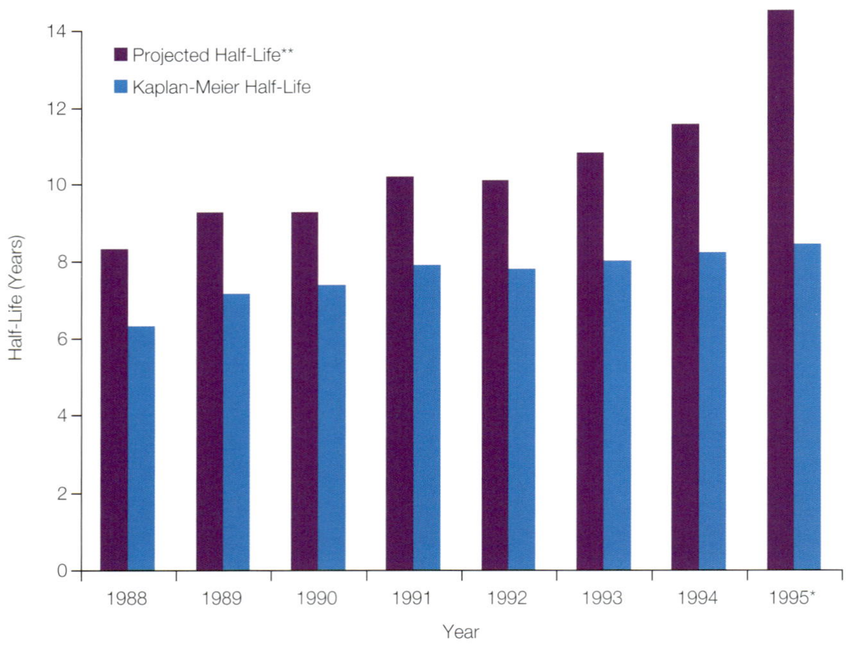

*Kaplan-Meier half-life based on time to 51% survival
** As published in Hariharan et al. (2000) NEJM 342:605

FIGURE 1-9. Projected versus actual half-lives. Source: Meier-Kreische, Schold, Kaplan (2004).

ALLOIMMUNE RESPONSE

It is now clear that a number of effector mechanisms, including the innate immune response, the humoral immune response, delayed type hypersensitivity, antibody dependent cytotoxicity and cytotoxic T cell responses, all contribute to the alloimmune response. The alloimmune response can be distinguished by the fact that it is associated with greater injury than is typical of immune responses against infectious pathogens. At the time of surgery, donor organs suffer ischemia-reperfusion injury, which creates a pro-inflammatory environment leading to a strong adaptive immune response. Secondary to injury caused by ischemia-reperfusion, donor graft cells undergo apoptosis, resulting in activation of macrophages and NK cells which are effectors of the innate immune system. The presence of pre-existing anti-donor Human Leukocyte Antigen (HLA) antibody can lead to activation of the complement system, resulting in deposits of C4d, a component of the complement cascade, along the blood vessels lining the graft (endothelium).

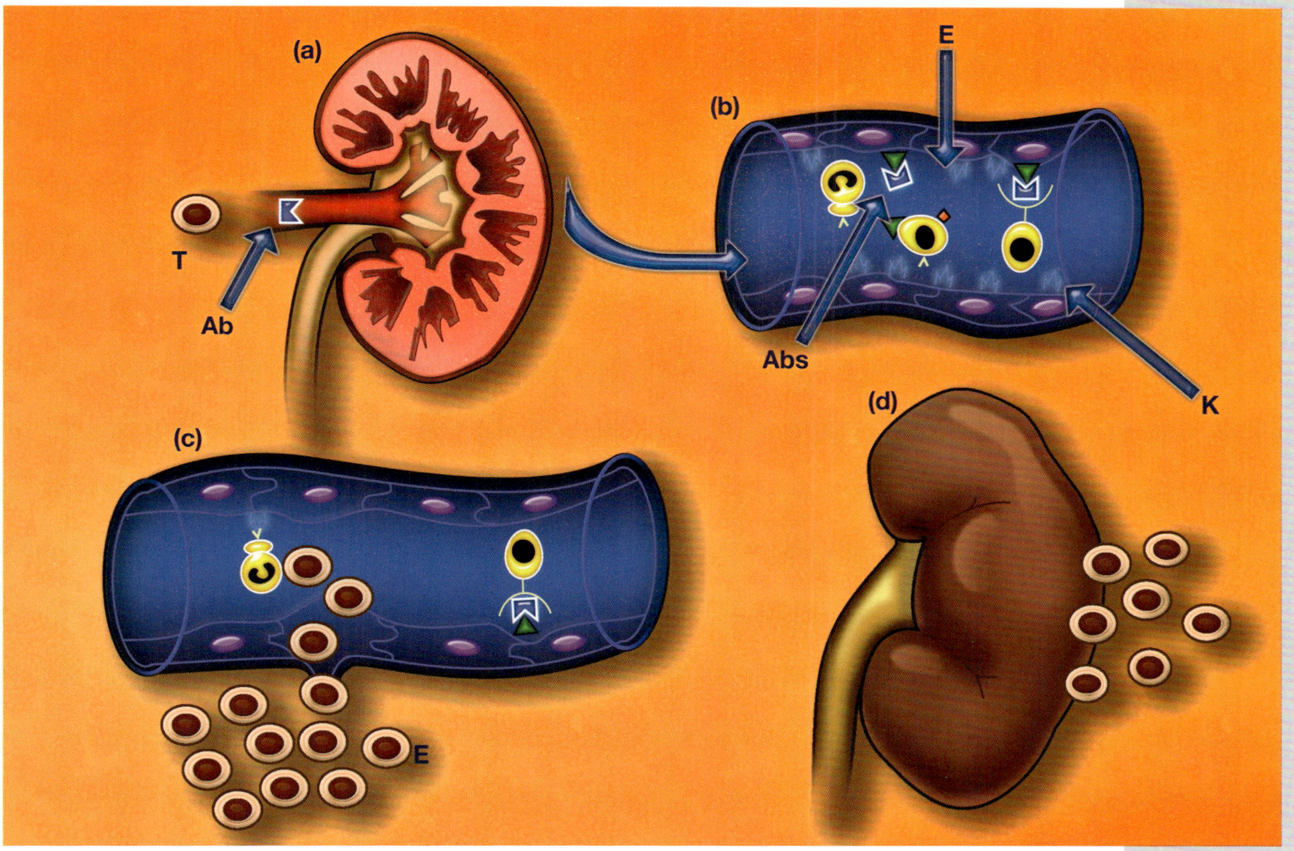

FIGURE 1-10. Mechanism of acute vascular rejection. Antibody binds to the endothelium followed by complement fixation and the influx of neutrophils and macrophages leading to vascular injury of the graft.

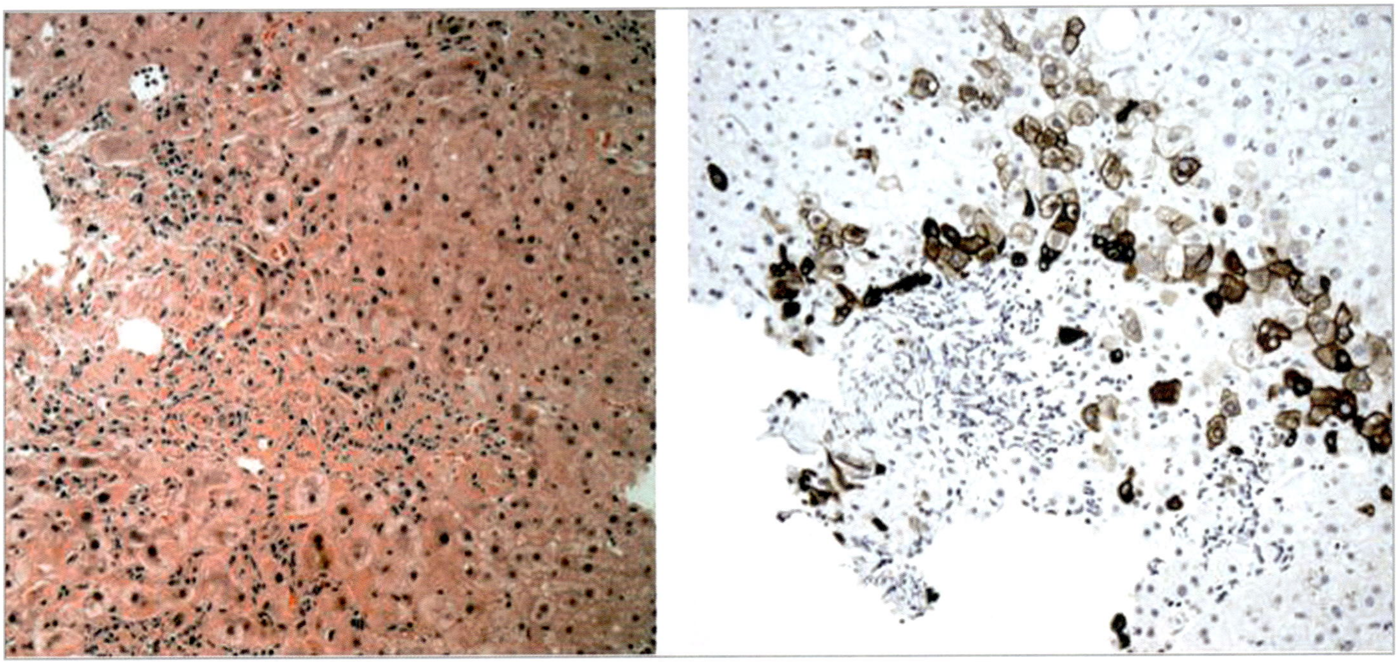

FIGURE 1-11. Chronic rejection in a liver allograft with bile duct loss and sparse inflammation (left panel H&E, 50x); same section stained with CK7 immunohistochemistry (right panel, 50x) showing absence of bile duct in portal tract but increased "intermediate" cells in the periportal zone.

MECHANISM OF ANTIBODY MEDIATED REJECTION

Antigen presenting cells (APCs) of both host and donor origin migrate to secondary lymphoid organs and present donor antigens directly or indirectly to naïve and central memory T cells as shown in Figure 1-12. T cells are then activated and undergo clonal expansion and differentiation. Donor antigen triggers T cell receptors (Signal 1) and co-stimulatory receptors, such as CD80 (B7-1) and CD86 (B7-2) (Signal 2) leading to activation of the calcium-calcineurin pathway, the mitogen activated protein kinase (MAP) pathway and protein kinase C pathway, which activates the transcription factors, nuclear factor of activated T cells (NFAT), activating protein 1 (AP-1) and NF-κB. This results in increased expression of the interleukin 2 receptor alpha chain (CD25) and interleukin 2, with subsequent expansion of long-lived memory T and B cells that serve to accelerate subsequent responses to the donor antigen (Signal 3). These memory cells are more resistant to the effects of modern immunosuppressive agents, representing a potent barrier to graft survival.

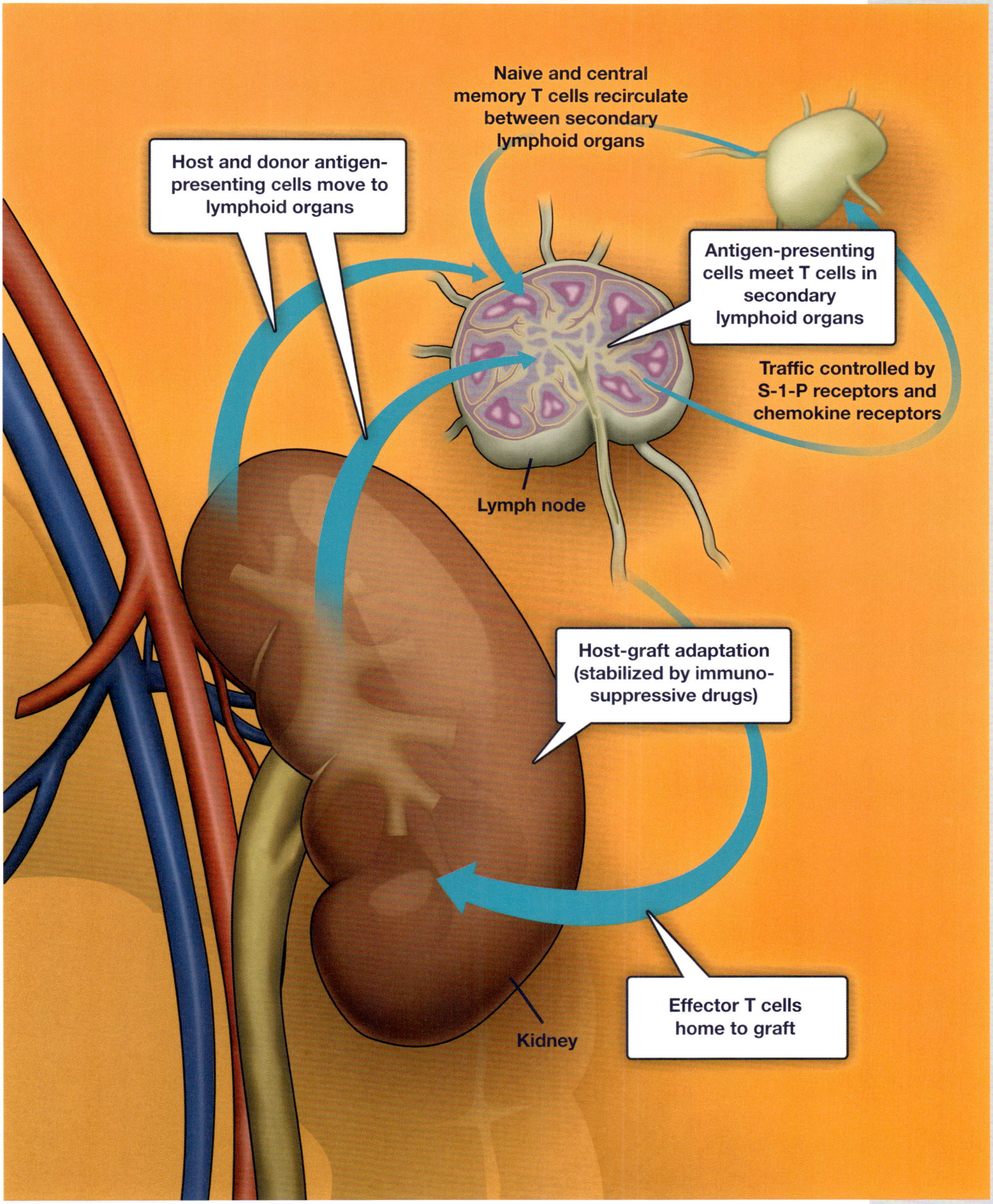

FIGURE 1-12. Steps in T cell mediated rejection. Adapted from Halloran (2004).

DONOR RECIPIENT MATCHING

The major barrier to allotransplantation is largely restricted to immune mediated recognition of Major Histocompatibility Complex (MHC) molecules expressed on donor tissue. Presently, it is standard practice to assign kidney and pancreas allografts on the basis of levels of mismatching of MHC alleles between donor and recipient. The practice is based upon historical studies showing that a measurable survival benefit is associated with a low level of mismatching between the donor and recipient MHC specificities, especially at the A, B and DR loci. MHC typing can be accomplished using a variety of methodologies including FLOW cytometry, real-time polymerase chain reaction (RTPCR) or serologic testing. Table 1-4 on the opposite page lists the genetic loci for MHC Class I and II. Figure 1-13 on the following page shows that graft survival rate decreases as the number of HLA mismatches increases.

TABLE 1-4. HLA Serology: Multiple Alleles May Exist for Each Locus

Class I MHC			Class II MHC		
HLA-A	HLA-B	HLA-C	HLA-DR	HLA-DQ	HLA-DP
A1	B7	Cw1	DR1	DQ2	DPw1
A2	B8	Cw2	DR3	DQ3	DPw2
A3	B13	Cw3	DR4	DQ4	DPw3
A11	B14	Cw4	DR7	DQ5	DPw4
A23	B15	Cw5	DR8	DQ6	DPw5
A24	B18	Cw6	DR9		DPw6
A25	B27	Cw7	DR10		
A26	B35	Cw8	DR11		
A29	B37		DR12		
A30	B38 (B16)		DR13		
A31	B39 (B16)		DR14		
A32	B40		DR15		
A33	B41		DR16		
A34	B42		DR51		
A36	B44 (B12)		DR52		
A43	B45 (B12)		DR53		
A66	B46				
A68	B47				
A69	B48				
A74	B49 (B21)				
	B50 (B21)				
	B51 (B5)				
	B52 (B5)				
	B53				
	B54 (B22)				
	B55 (B22)				
	B56 (B22)				
	B57 (B17)				
	B58 (B17)				
	B59				
	B67				
	B73				
	B78				

w = workshop assignments when serologic assignments are imprecise.

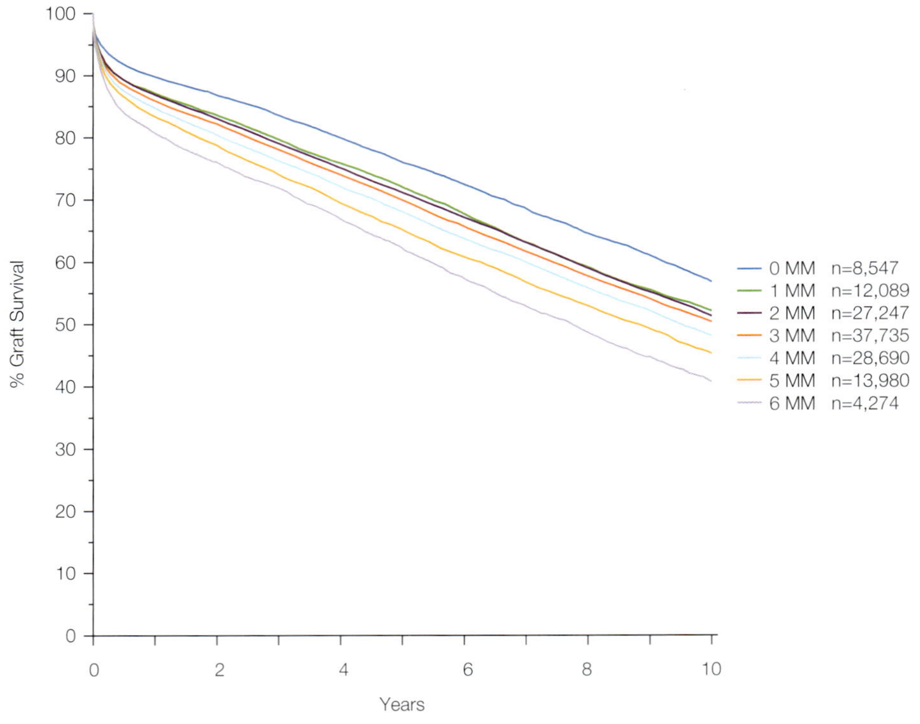

FIGURE 1-13. HLA-A+B+DR Mismatches, Deceased Donor, First Kidney Transplants 1985-2007. Data from Collaborative Transplant Study-K-21101-February 2009.

Previous encounters with cells that possess MHC antigens, such as occurs following blood transfusion, pregnancy or a previous transplant, can result in long-lived memory B cells and persistence of anti MHC-antibody. If an organ is transplanted into an individual who has pre-existing antibody to the donor MHC, the antibody will bind to the endothelium of the donor organ, activate complement and coagulation, resulting in immediate loss of the graft. In cross-matching procedures, donor T and B cells are incubated with serum from the prospective recipient to test for binding that would indicate the presence of these antibodies. This pre-transplant cross-matching is now done routinely for recipients of kidney and pancreas allografts and is also performed selectively on recipients of hearts and lungs. Positive cross-matches preclude transplantation and the organ would be assigned to an alternative recipient.

Approaches to decrease or eliminate these antibodies through desensitization protocols are now being studied to allow these pre-sensitized patients to undergo allotransplantation as shown below in Figure 1-14 and Table 1-5.

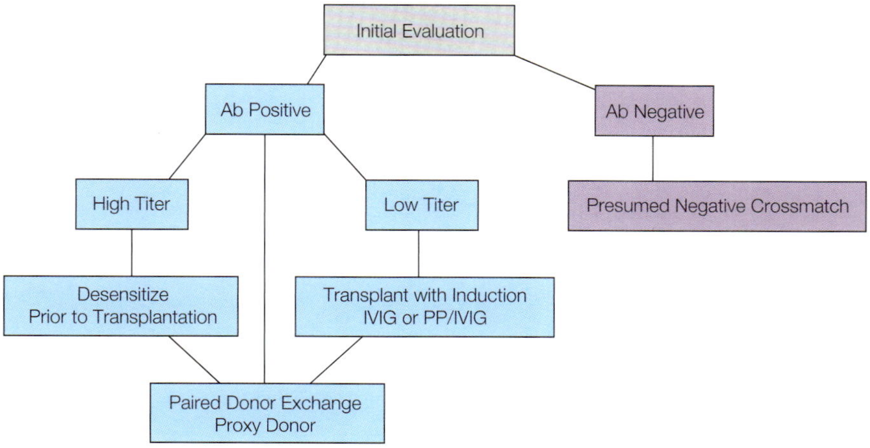

FIGURE 1-14. Laboratory approaches for evaluating the sensitized: Ab = HLA alloantibody; PP=plasmapheresis; IVIG=intravenous immune globulin. Adapted from Gebel and Bray (2008).

TABLE 1-5. Approaches for Transplanting the Sensitized Patient

Biological	Pharmacological
Identical Sibling	Transplanting across a Positive crossmatch – Thymoglobulin +/- IVIG – ALG – Rituximab – Campath-1
Negative Crossmatch – Compatible living donor – Emory Algorithm – HLA Matchmaker/Acceptable Mismatch Program – Paired Donor Exchange – Proxy donation	Desensitization Protocols – IVIG (high dose) – PP/IVIG (low dose)

ALG=antilymphocyte globulin; IVIG=intravenous immune globulin; PP=plasma-pheresis.
Adapted from Gebel and Bray (2008).

USEFUL WEBSITES

Scientific Registry of Transplant Recipients (SRTR) supports the ongoing evaluation of scientific and clinical status of solid organ transplantation in the United States. www.ustransplant.org

United Network for Organ Sharing (UNOS) facilitates organ sharing among the transplant centers in the United States. www.unos.org

Eurotransplant International Foundation facilitates organ procurement among several European countries. www.eurotransplant.nl

Collaborative Transplant Study (CTS) based in Germany is the largest international voluntary study group with over 400 transplant centers in 45 countries. www.ctstransplant.org

The American Society of Transplantation (AST) is an international organization of transplant professionals dedicated to advancing the field of transplantation through a variety of means to improve patient care. www.a-s-t.org

BIBLIOGRAPHY FOR CHAPTER 1

Meier-Kriesche HU, Schold JD, Kaplan B. Long term renal allograft survival: Have we made significant progress or is it time to rethink our analytic and therapeutic strategies? Am J Transplant. 2004;4:1289-95.

Murphy K, Travers P, Walport M. Janeway's Immunology, 7th Edition. 2008. Chapter 14, Garland Science Taylor and Francis Group, Mortimer House, London, UK.

Halloran, PF. Immunosuppressive drugs for kidney transplantation. N Engl J Med. 2004;351:2715-29.

Vincenti F and Kirk AD. What's next in the pipeline. Am J Transplant. 2008;8:1972-81.

Gebel HM and Bray RA. Approaches for transplanting the sensitized patient: biology versus pharmacology. Nephrol Dial Transplant. 2008;2454-7.

Kahan BD. Cyclosporine. N Engl J Med. 1989;321:1725-38.

Ojo AO, Held PJ, Port FK, Wolfe RA, Leichtman AB, Young EW, Arndorfer J, Christensen L, Merion RM. Chronic renal failure after transplantation of a nonrenal organ. N Engl J Med. 2003;349:931-40.

Chadban S, Morris R, Hirsch HH, Bunnapradist S, Arns W, Budde K. Immunosuppression in renal transplantation: some aspects for the modern era. Transplantation Reviews. 2008;22:241-251.

Flechner SM, Kobashigawa J, Klintmalm G. Calcineurin inhibitor sparing regimens in solid organ transplantation: focus on improving renal function and nephrotoxicity. Clin Transplant. 2008;22:1-15.

Ojo AO, Meier-Kriesche HU, Hanson JA et.al. Mycophenolate mofetil reduces late renal allograft loss independent of acute rejection. Transplantation 2000;69:2405-9.

Webster AC, Lee VW, Chapman JR et al. Target of rapamycin inhibitors (sirolimus and everolimus) for primary immunosuppression of kidney transplant recipients: a systematic review and meta-analysis of randomized trials. Transplantation. 2006; 81:1234-48.

Nankivell BJ, Borrows RJ, Fung CLS et.al. Evolution and pathophysiology of renal-transplant glomulerosclerosis. Transplantation. 2004;78:461-8.

McCullough KP, Keith DS, Meyer KH et al. Kidney and pancreas transplantation in the United States, 1998-2007: Access for patients with diabetes and end-stage renal disease. Am J Transplant. 2009;9:894-906.

Wolfe RA, Merion RM, Roys EC, Port FK. Trends in organ donation and transplantation in the United States, 1998-2007. Am J Transplant. 2009;9:869-78.

Latta P, Ricordi C, Scharp D. Paul E. Lacy, MD, PhD February 7, 1924 to February 15, 2005. Special Article. Am J Transplant. 2005;5:976-7.

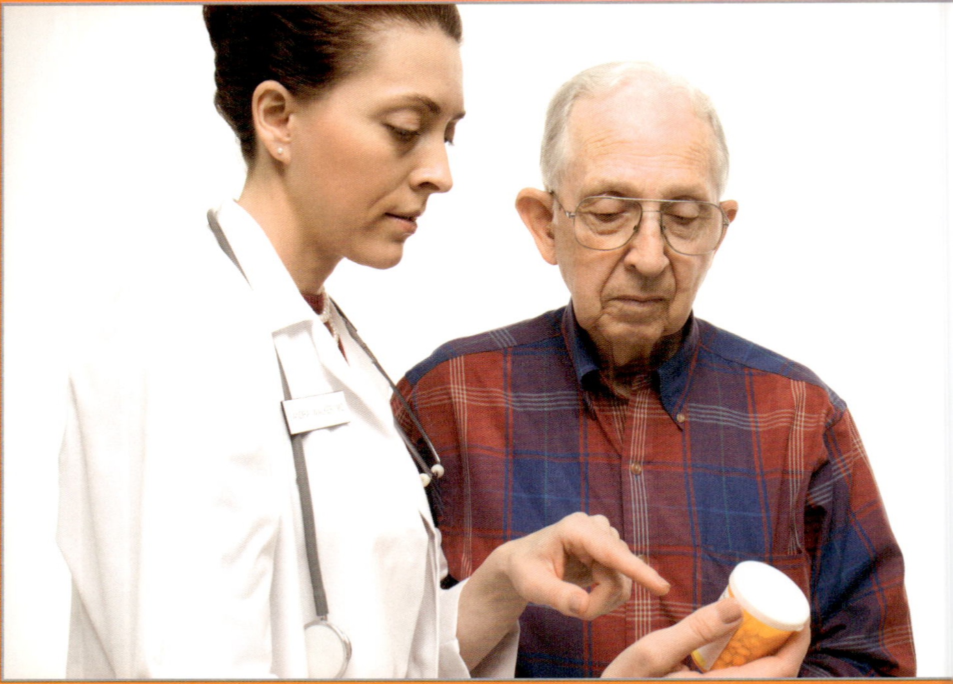

CHAPTER 2 CONTENTS

INTRODUCTION TO IMMUNOSUPPRESSION AND IMMUNOSUPPRESSIVE DRUGS

Immunosuppression is defined as the prevention or interference with the development of the normal immunologic response. Immunosuppression can occur through disease, such as HIV, which kills T cells, as well as chemicals via drugs, or through biological compounds such as therapeutic antibodies. The immune response protects the human body against foreign insults, be they bacteria, viruses or cancer. The immune system also recognizes an allograft as a foreign body and will mount a vigorous immune response against the allograft in an attempt to destroy it. In order for a person to suppress this normal response against an allograft they need to take an immunosuppressive agent(s). Immunosuppression is necessary to prevent destruction of the graft by the immune system of the recipient (host).

Recognition of foreign antigens by the T cell occurs through the presentation of the foreign antigen cognate peptides by the MHC complex present on the surface of an Antigen Presenting Cell (APC). These peptide antigens can be derived from infectious agents invading the host and can also be derived from the donor allograft organ. As shown below in Figure 2-1 and on the adjacent page in Figure 2-2, the presentation of foreign antigens by the APC to the T cell triggers activation and replication of the T cell through three specific signals.

Signal 1 ⟶ APC:MHC-antigen complex binds to the T cell:CD3 receptor

Signal 2 ⟶ APC:CD80, 86 binds to the T cell:CD28 receptor

Signal 1
\+
Signal 2 ⟶ T cell: Activation of signal transduction pathways leading to synthesis of IL-2, CD154, and CD25 (co-stimulation)

Signal 3 ⟶ T cell: Synthesis of IL-2, CD154, and CD25 plus other cytokines trigger T cell proliferation

FIGURE 2-1. Three signals required for T cell proliferation.

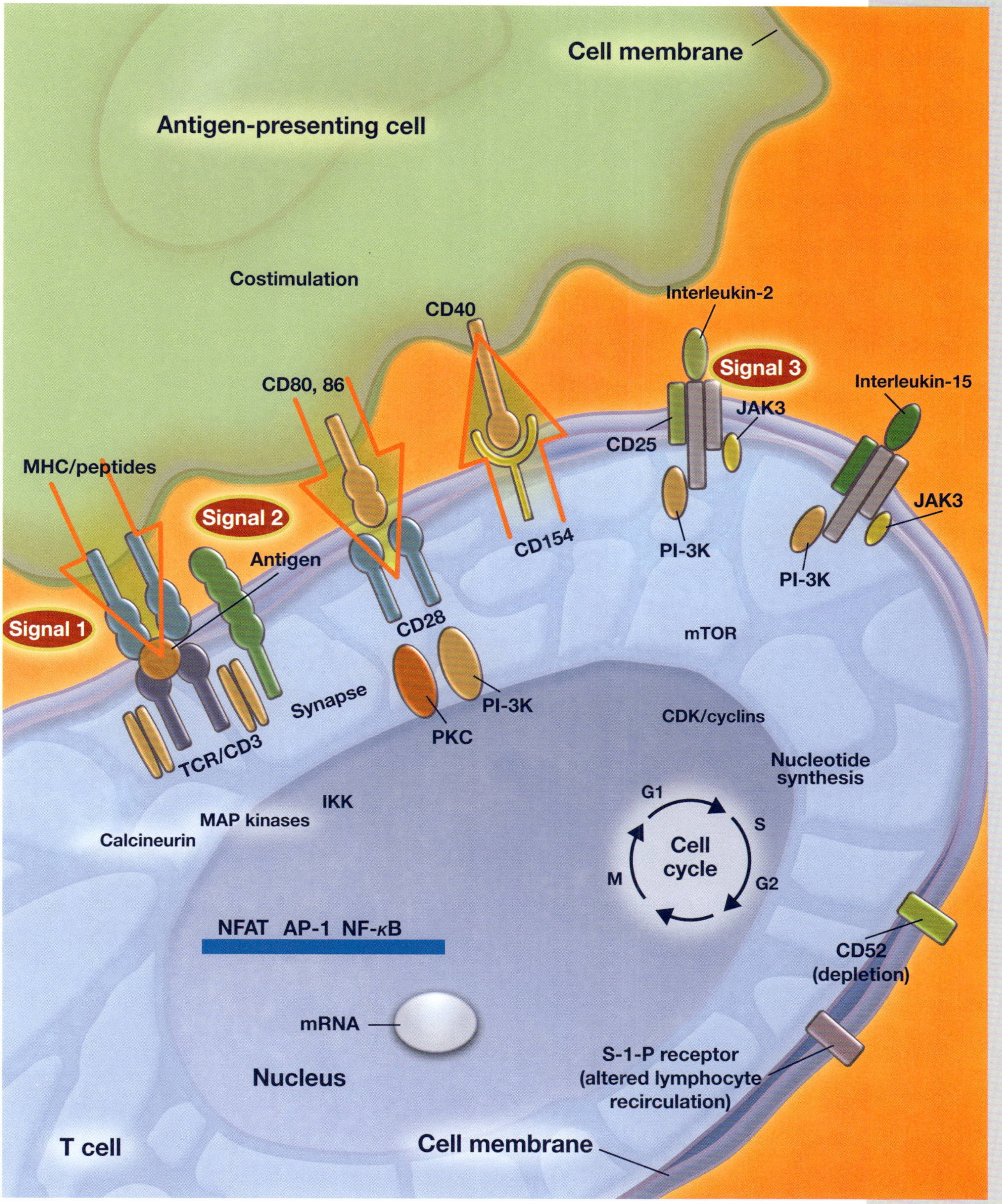

FIGURE 2-2. Schematic representation of the interaction between an APC and T cell in lymphoid tissue. Adapted from Halloran (2004).

As shown in Figure 2-3, the interaction of the APC:MHC-antigen complex with the T cell:CD3 receptor (Signal 1) and APC:CD80, 86 with T cell:CD28 receptor (Signal 2) activates three signal transduction pathways. Activation of the calcium-calcineurin pathway, the mitogen activated protein (MAP) kinase pathway, and the nuclear factor-κB (NF-κB) pathway then activates the transcription factors nuclear factor of activated T cells (NFAT), activating protein 1 (AP-1) and NF-κB, respectively. This results in mRNA synthesis and expression of IL-2, CD154 (activates APCs), and CD25. IL-2 binds to the IL-2 receptor (CD25) present on the T cell (Signal 3) and, in collaboration with other cytokines, activation of the mammalian target of rapamycin (mTOR) pathway occurs, leading to activation of the cell cycle. Upon transduction by Signal 3, quiescent T cells in the G_0 resting phase of the cell cycle move into G_1 phase, the growing phase, in preparation for DNA synthesis. Lymphocyte proliferation requires the *de novo* synthesis of purine and pyrimidine nucleotides for DNA replication, which begins during G_1 and continues through S phase, the DNA synthesis phase, when the chromosomes of the cell are duplicated. Once the chromosomes are duplicated in S phase the T cell enters the G_2 phase and continues to grow in preparation for cell division, which occurs during the M or mitotic phase of the cell cycle. If continued antigenic stimulation by APCs occurs the T cells enter G_1 phase again and each subsequent turn of the cell cycle results in a rapid clonal expansion of T cells capable of recognizing the cognate foreign antigen that stimulated their expansion.

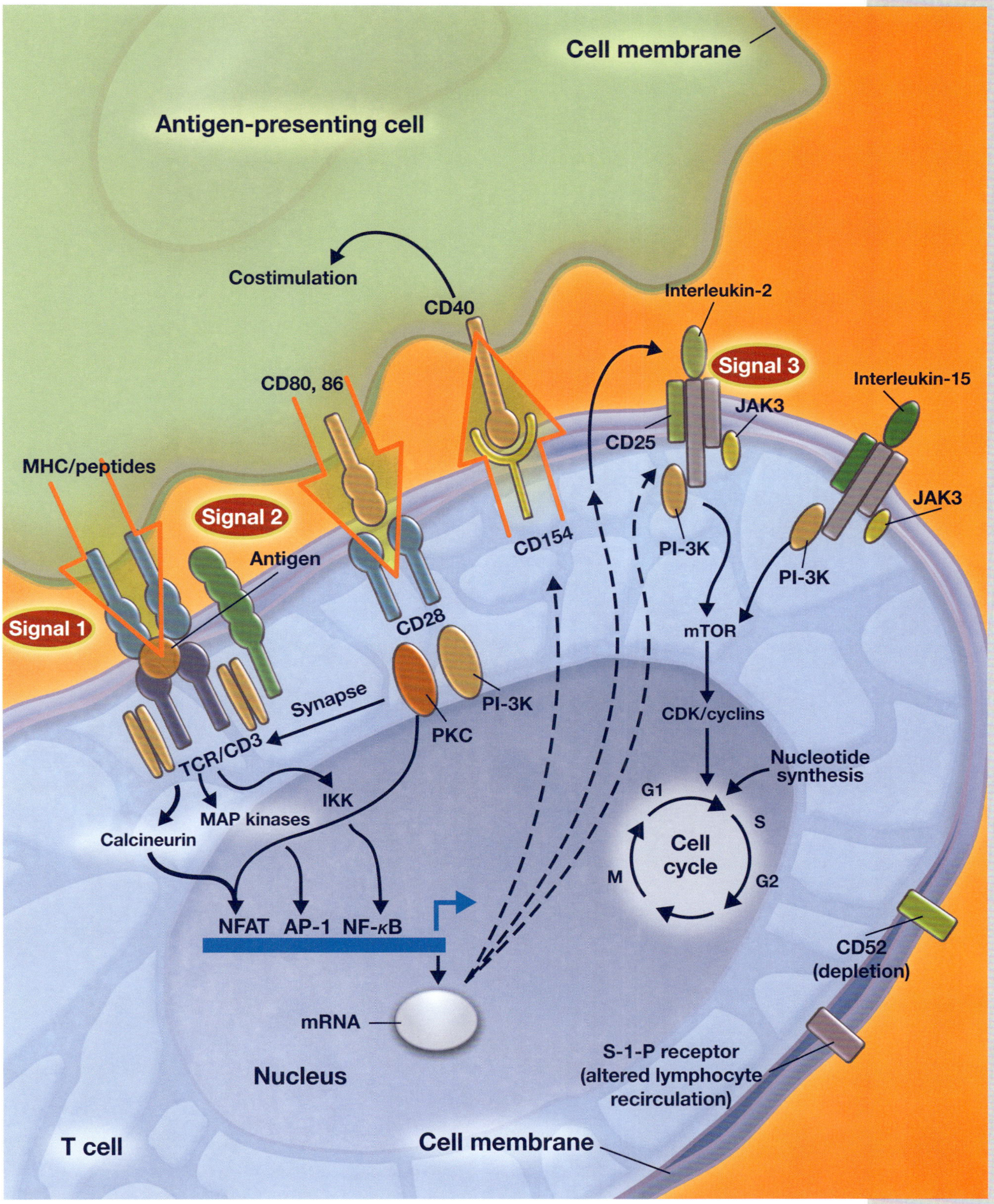

FIGURE 2-3. Presentation of a foreign antigen by an APC to a T cell activates Signal 1, Signal 2, and Signal 3 leading to T cell proliferation. Adapted from Halloran (2004).

There have been tremendous advances in immunosuppression over the past 30 years which have led to a marked improvement in patient and graft survival. As shown in Figure 2-4, the initial development of steroid therapy, azathioprine (AZA), and anti-lymphocyte antisera as immunosuppressive agents opened the door to solid organ transplantation. The discovery of the calcineurin inhibitor cyclosporine (CsA, CsA-ME) revolutionized the field and significantly increased both patient and graft survival. The subsequent development of additional biological (anti-thymocyte globulin) and chemical (tacrolimus [TAC], sirolimus [RAPA], everolimus [SDZ-RAD], mycophenolate mofetil [MMF]) immunosuppressive agents has significantly reduced the problem of acute rejection which plagued the early years of transplantation.

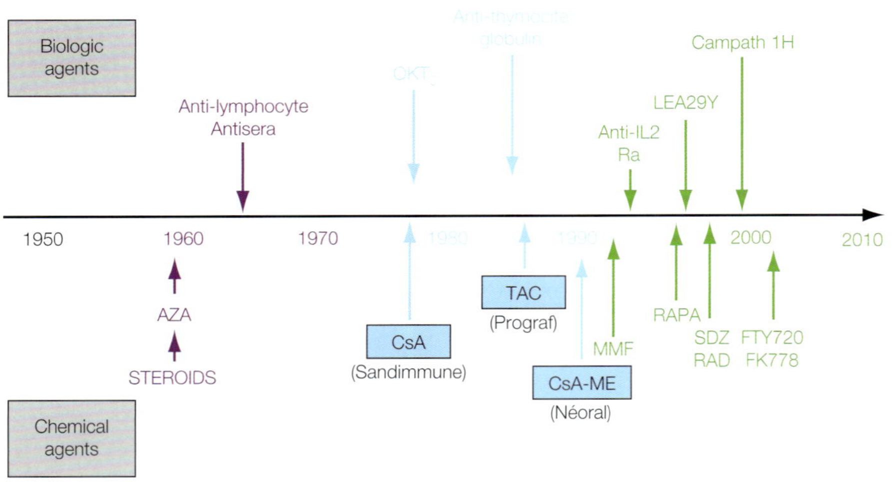

FIGURE 2-4. Timeline for development of immunosuppressive agents.

Immunosuppression can be achieved by depleting lymphocytes, diverting lymphocyte traffic or blocking lymphocyte response pathways as shown in Figure 2-5 on the adjacent page. Immunosuppression, which will be discussed below in detail, consists of a combination of drugs that are used to prevent allograft rejection. Most drugs currently available are designed to block lymphocyte activation and proliferation. Induction immunosuppression refers to the use of immunosuppression in the immediate peri-transplant period. Biological agents, including polyclonal anti-lymphocyte globulin, anti-CD25 (basiliximab) or anti-CD52 (alemtuzumab) in combination with high doses of corticosteroids are currently being used as induction agents.

Tacrolimus and cyclosporine, the current mainstays of maintenance immunosuppression, bind to cytoplasmic proteins called immunophilins, to form a complex that blocks the phosphatase activity of calcineurin. This prevents formation and release of the growth factor IL-2. Anti-proliferative agents, including azathioprine and mycophenolic acid, a noncompetitive inhibitor of inosine monophosphate dehydrogenase, have played a pivotal role in immunosuppressive regimens since the original demonstration of their efficacy by Calne. The mTOR inhibitors, sirolimus and everolimus inhibit activation of an S6 kinase that prevents progression of the cell cycle from G_1 to the S phase, blocking T cell proliferation. Newer agents being studied include Belatacept, a monoclonal antibody that blocks binding of CD28 with CD80 or CD86 and prevents the co-stimulation signal normally provided through this pathway, and AEB071, a protein kinase C inhibitor. Potentially, either could substitute for cyclosporine or tacrolimus, either alone or in combination with mycophenolic acid, mTOR inhibitors and steroids.

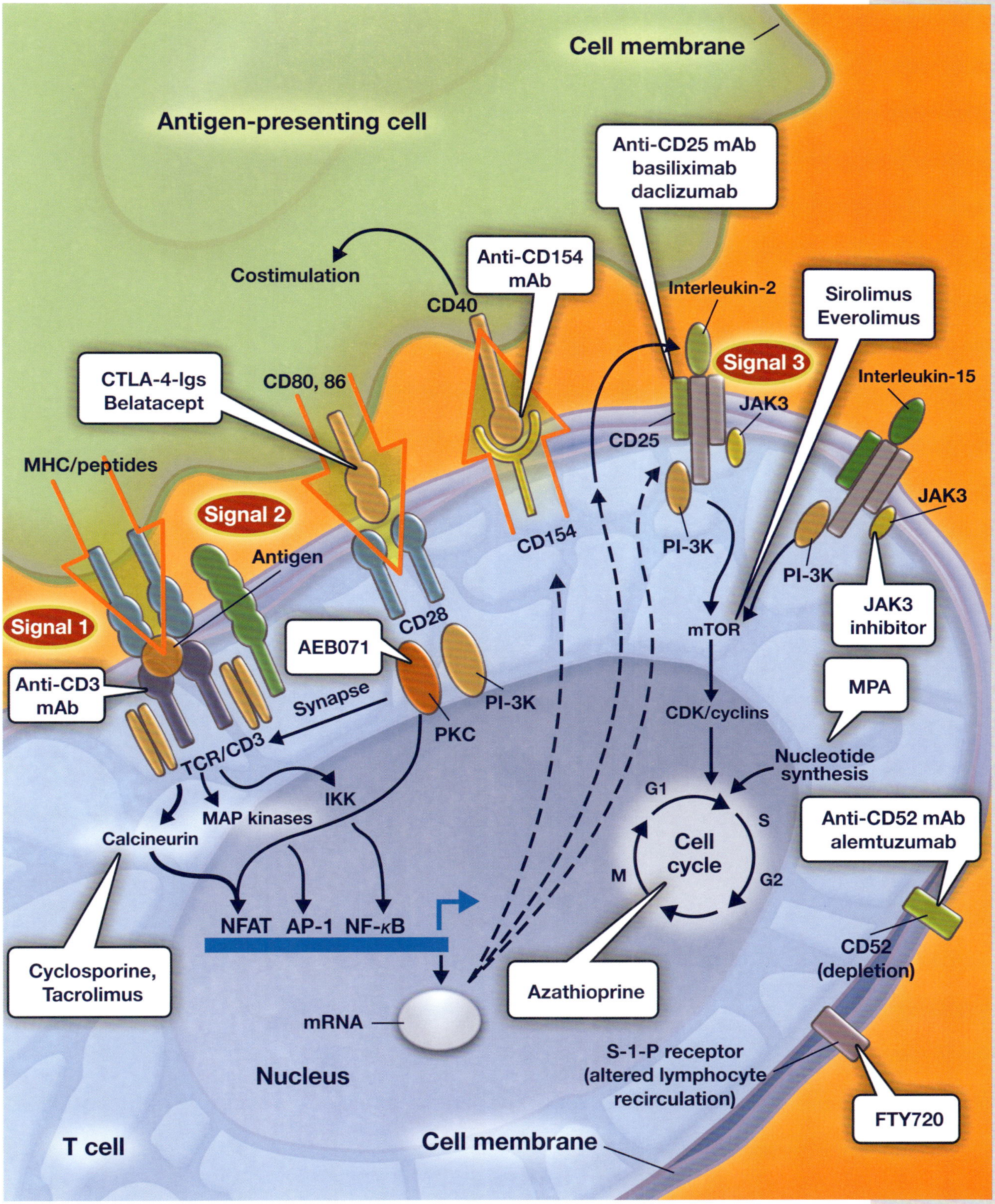

FIGURE 2-5. Site of action of immunosuppressive drugs. Adapted from Halloran (2004).

OPTIMIZING IMMUNOSUPPRESSION

Immunosuppression is accomplished through the use of a dosed regimen. An ideal combination of drugs prevents the development of acute rejection but does not induce so much immunosuppression that the patient is at increased risk for infection, malignancy, toxicity, and other complications of the immunosuppressive drugs.

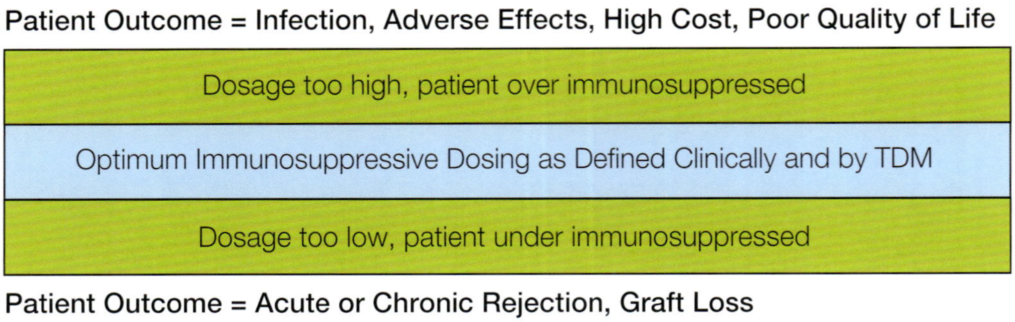

FIGURE 2-6. Balance of immunosuppression.

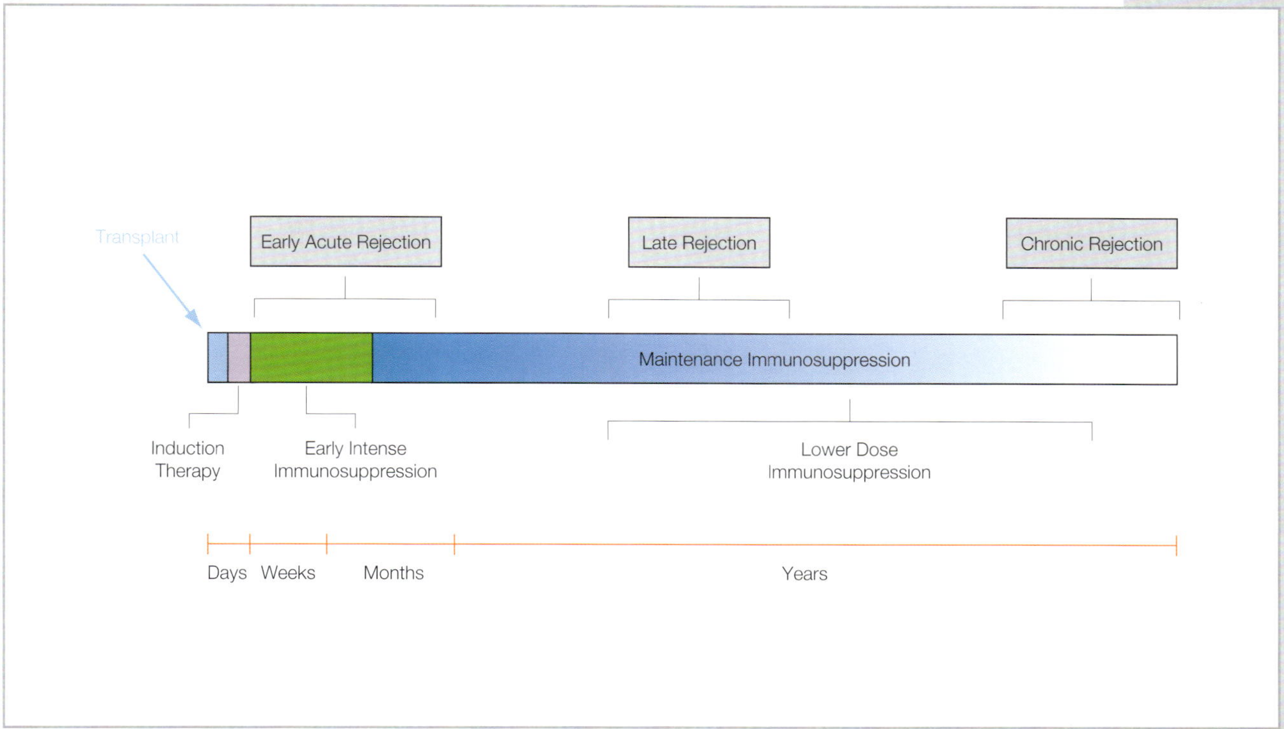

FIGURE 2-7. Phases of transplantation.

INDUCTION THERAPY

Induction therapy is the use of potent immunosuppressive antibodies given intravenously at the time of transplantation to rapidly achieve a state of immunosuppression. The rationale for induction immunosuppression is to provide intense immunosuppression during the early post-transplant period, when the risk of acute rejection is highest. Induction therapy regimens vary by organ type and are used less frequently in liver transplant recipients, in whom an episode of acute rejection is not predictive of long-term outcomes. The use of this therapy decreases the risk of acute cellular rejection and the impact of rejection on long-term outcome. An episode of rejection is an important predictor of an increased risk of graft loss in all other solid organ transplant recipients. In liver transplant recipients induction therapy is generally used in patients with renal failure, in whom the introduction of calcineurin inhibitors is delayed.

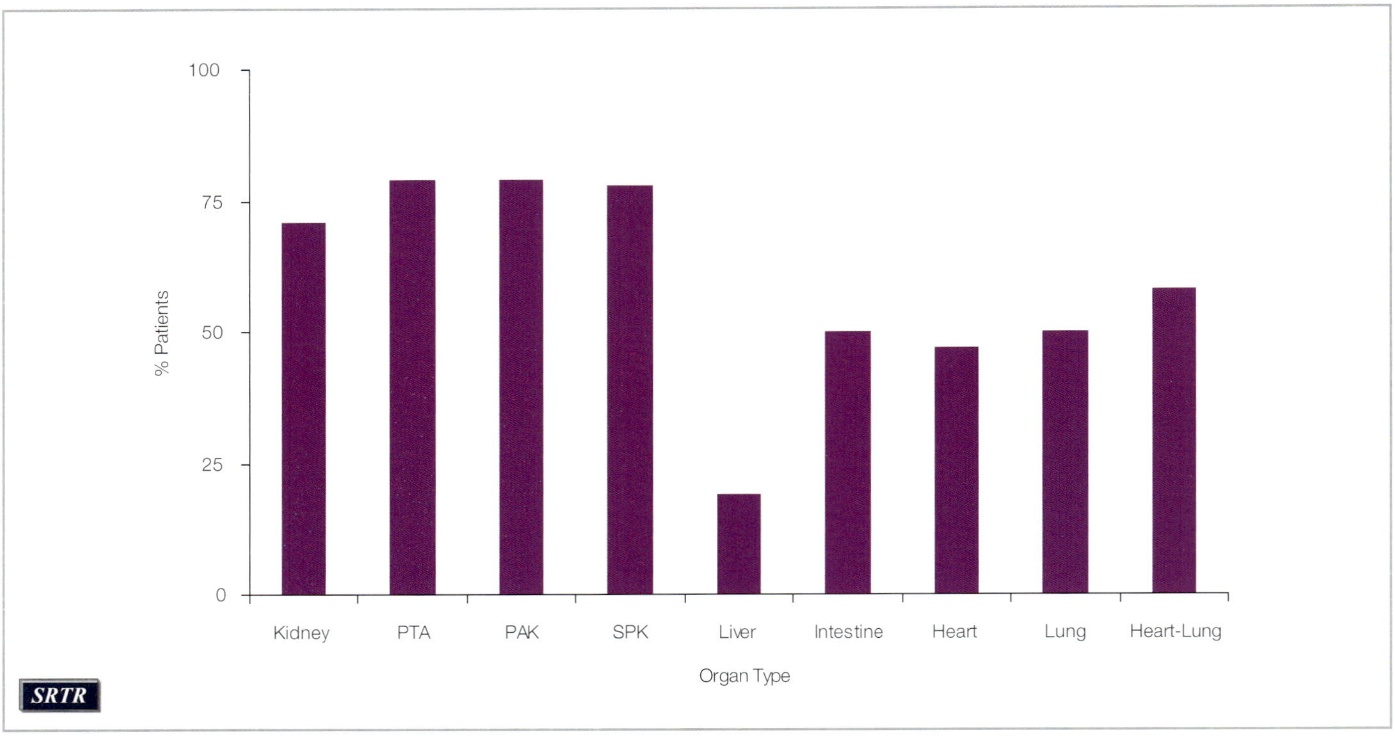

FIGURE 2-8. Distribution of induction therapy by organ type. PTA: Pancreas Transplant alone; PAK: Pancreas After Kidney; SPK: Simultaneous Pancreas-Kidney. Adapted from: 2005 OPTN/SRTR Annual Report, 1997-2006. HHS/HRSA/HSB/DOT. Table 1.9.

As shown in Figure 2-8, induction therapy is most common in kidney and pancreas allograft recipients and least common in liver allograft recipients. Figure 2-9 shows the use of induction agents following kidney transplantation. Thymoglobulin, a potent T cell depletion agent, is the most common induction agent. Campath-1H (alemtuzumab), which is indicated for the treatment of B cell chronic lymphocytic leukemia, has seen increasing usage as an induction agent. Table 2-1 describes the commonly used induction agents and their mechanisms of action.

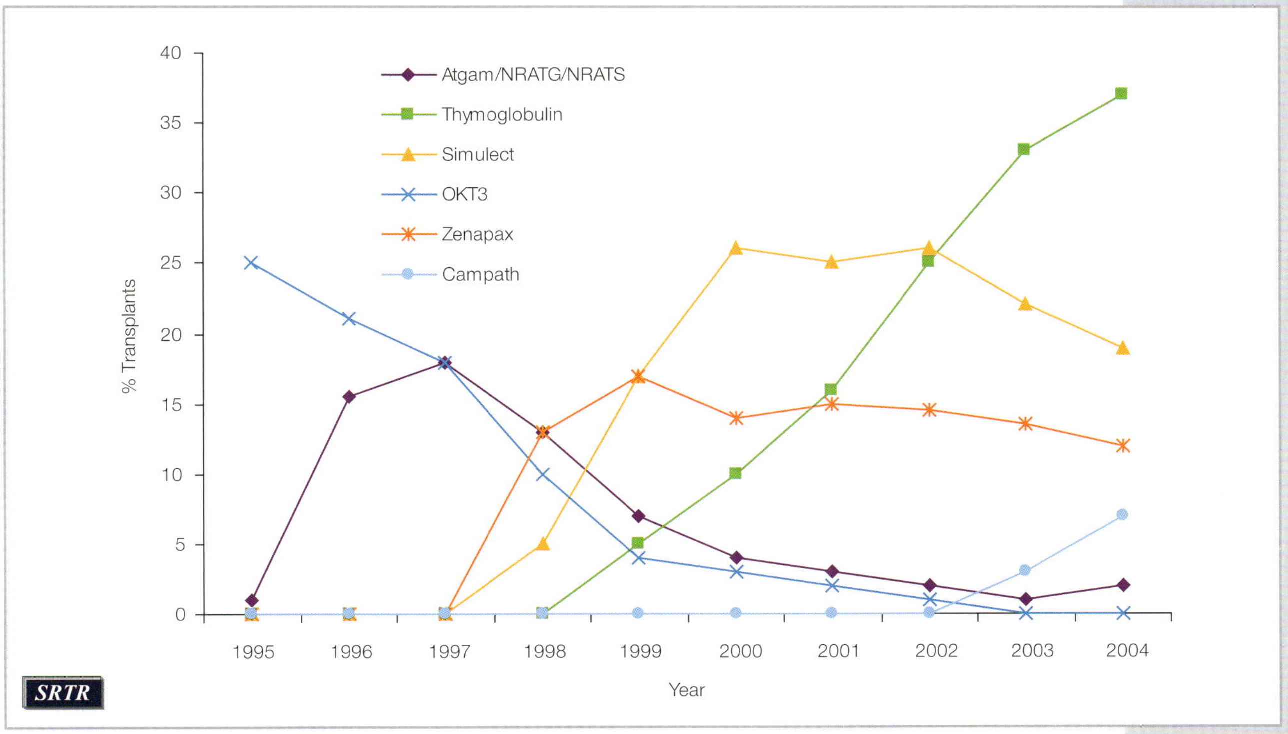

FIGURE 2-9. Immunosuppression agents used for induction in kidney transplantation, 1995-2004. Adapted from: 2005 OPTN/SRTR Annual Report, 1997-2006. HHS/HRSA/HSB/DOT. Table 5.6a and Meier-Kriesche (2006) et al.

TABLE 2-1. Induction Agents and Mechanisms of Action

Drug	Target	Mechanism of Action
OKT3	anti-CD3	T cell antigen recognition antagonist
Zenapax® (daclizumab)	anti-CD25	IL-2 receptor antagonist
Simulect® (basiliximab)	anti-CD25	IL-2 receptor antagonist
Campath-1H® (alemtuzumab)	anti-CD52	T cell depletion
Thymoglobulin® (thymocyte globulin)	T cell antigens	T cell depletion
Atgam/NRATG/NRATS	T cell antigens	T cell depletion

MAINTENANCE THERAPY

Maintenance therapy is the use of orally administered immunosuppressive drugs after transplantation to maintain adequate immunosuppression and prevent rejection.

The two main drugs used in maintenance immunosuppression therapy are the calcineurin inhibitors (CNIs) tacrolimus and cyclosporine. Tacrolimus has now become the CNI of choice for maintenance therapy in most solid organ transplants, with the exception of heart allografts as shown in Figure 2-10. These drugs can be used alone or, more often, they are used in conjunction with steroids and other co-therapeutic drugs such as azathioprine or mycophenolic acid. The mTOR inhibitors sirolimus and everolimus may also be used in conjunction with tacrolimus or cyclosporine, but tacrolimus and cyclosporine have the same mechanism of action and are not used together. A list of maintenance immunosuppressive agents and their mechanism of action is shown in Table 2-2 and their chemical structures are shown in Figures 2-11, 2-12, 2-13, 2-14, 2-15, and 2-16. Figure 2-17 summarizes the "immunosuppressant cocktail" that is commonly used to achieve adequate maintenance immunosuppression in transplant recipients. A combination or "cocktail" of drugs is used to inhibit the different signal transduction pathways (Signals 1-3) discussed earlier that are required for T cell proliferation and concomitant graft rejection.

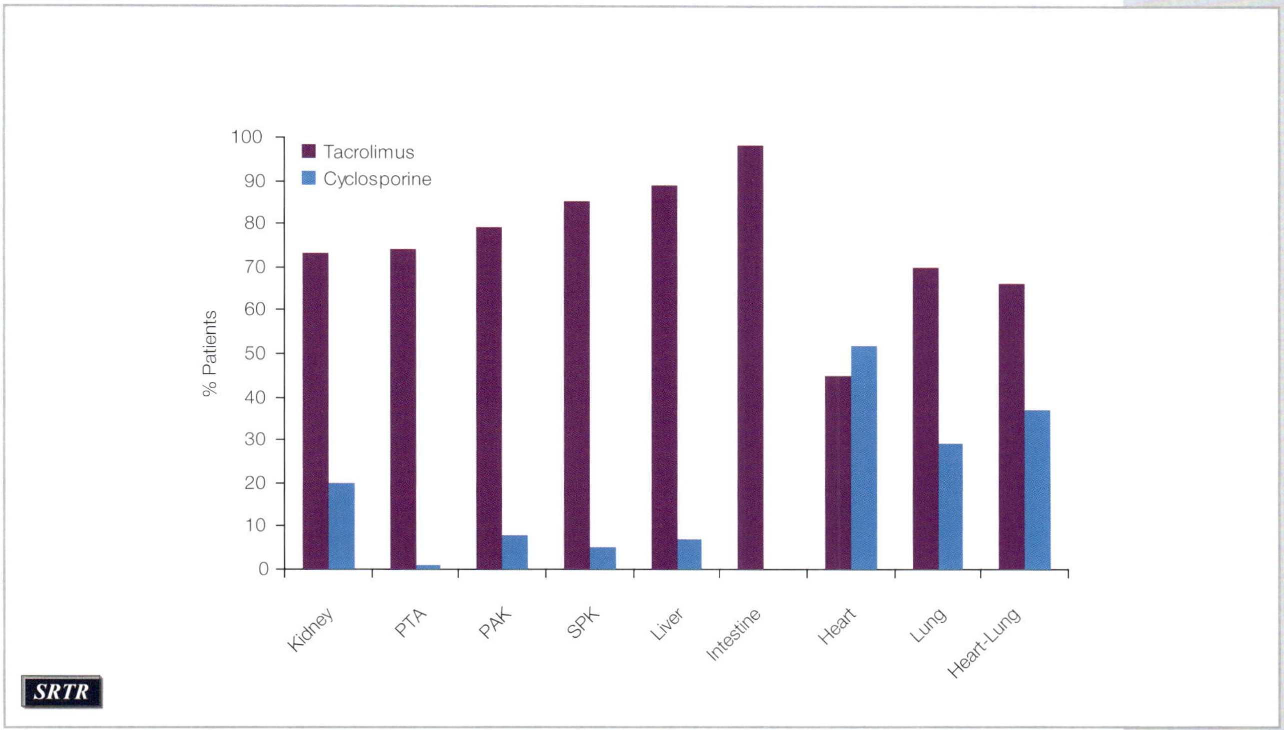

FIGURE 2-10. Distribution of maintenance CNI therapy by organ type. PTA: Pancreas Transplant alone; PAK: Pancreas After Kidney; SPK: Simultaneous Pancreas-Kidney. Adapted from: 2005 OPTN/SRTR Annual Report, 1997-2006. HHS/HRSA/HSB/DOT. Table 1.9.

TABLE 2-2. Maintenance Therapeutic Agents and Mechanisms of Action

Drug	Target	Mechanism of Action
Prograf®, Advagraf®, Tacrobell® (Tacrolimus)	CNI	Blocks IL-2 synthesis
Neoral®, Sandimmune® (Cyclosporine)	CNI	Blocks IL-2 synthesis
Rapamune® (Sirolimus)	mTOR	Blocks IL-2 driven T cell proliferation
Certican® (Everolimus)	mTOR	Blocks IL-2 driven T cell proliferation
Cellcept® (Mycophenolate mofetil, MMF)	Purine synthesis	Blocks B and T cell proliferation
Myfortic® (Enteric-coated mycophenolate sodium)	Purine synthesis	Blocks B and T cell proliferation
Imuran® (Azathioprine)	Purine synthesis	Blocks B and T cell proliferation

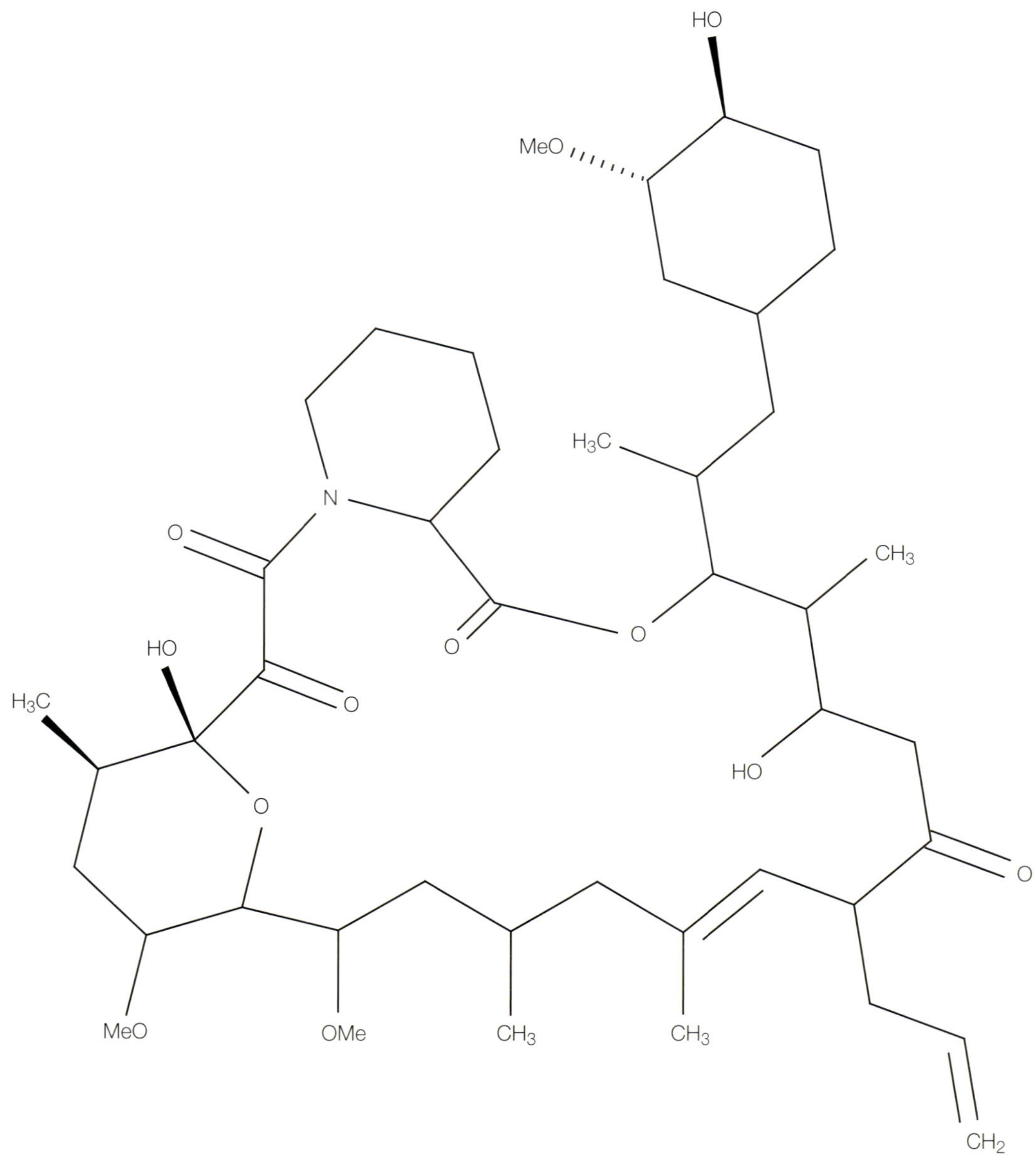

FIGURE 2-11. Chemical structure of tacrolimus, calcineurin inhibitor.

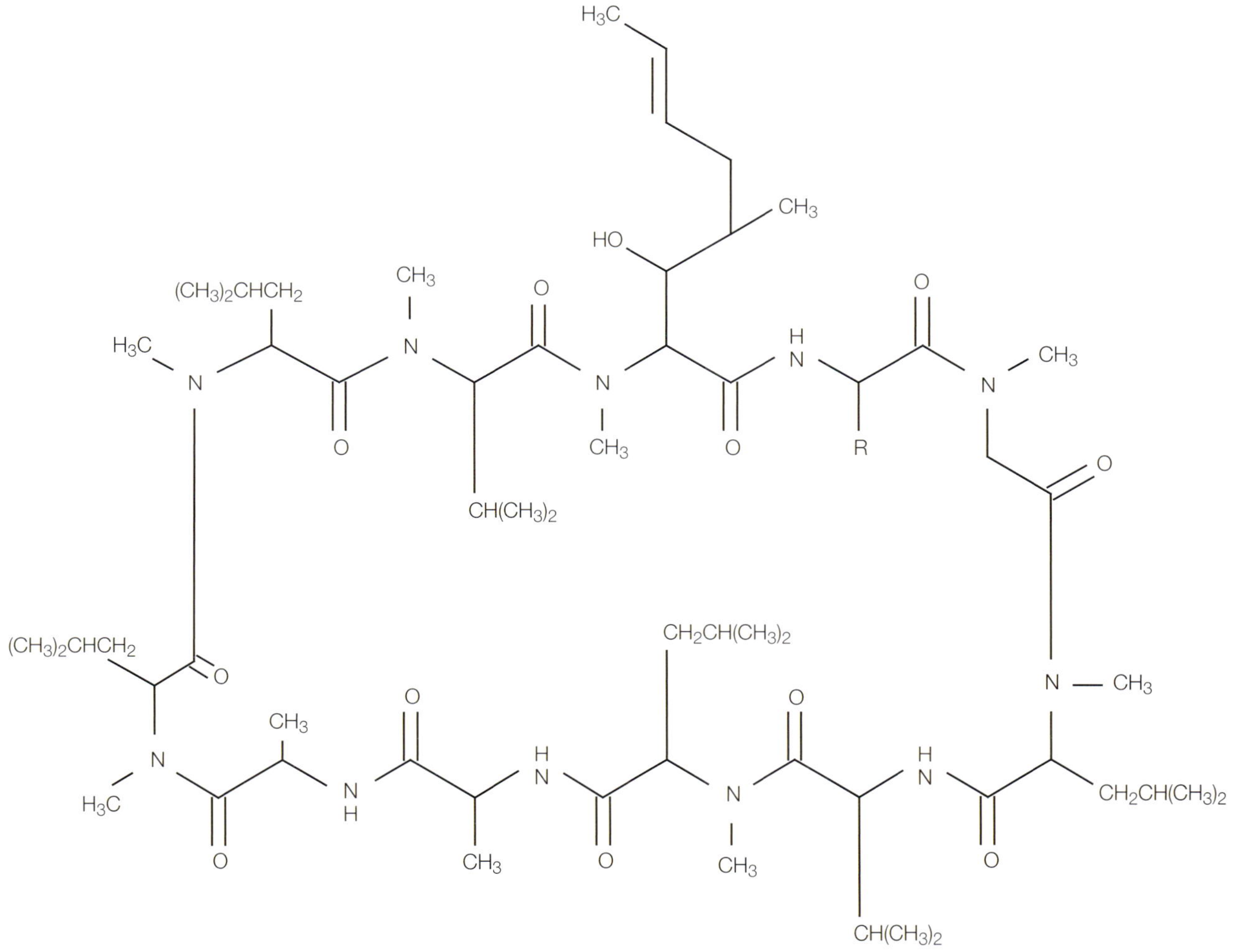

FIGURE 2-12. Chemical structure of cyclosporine, calcineurin inhibitor.

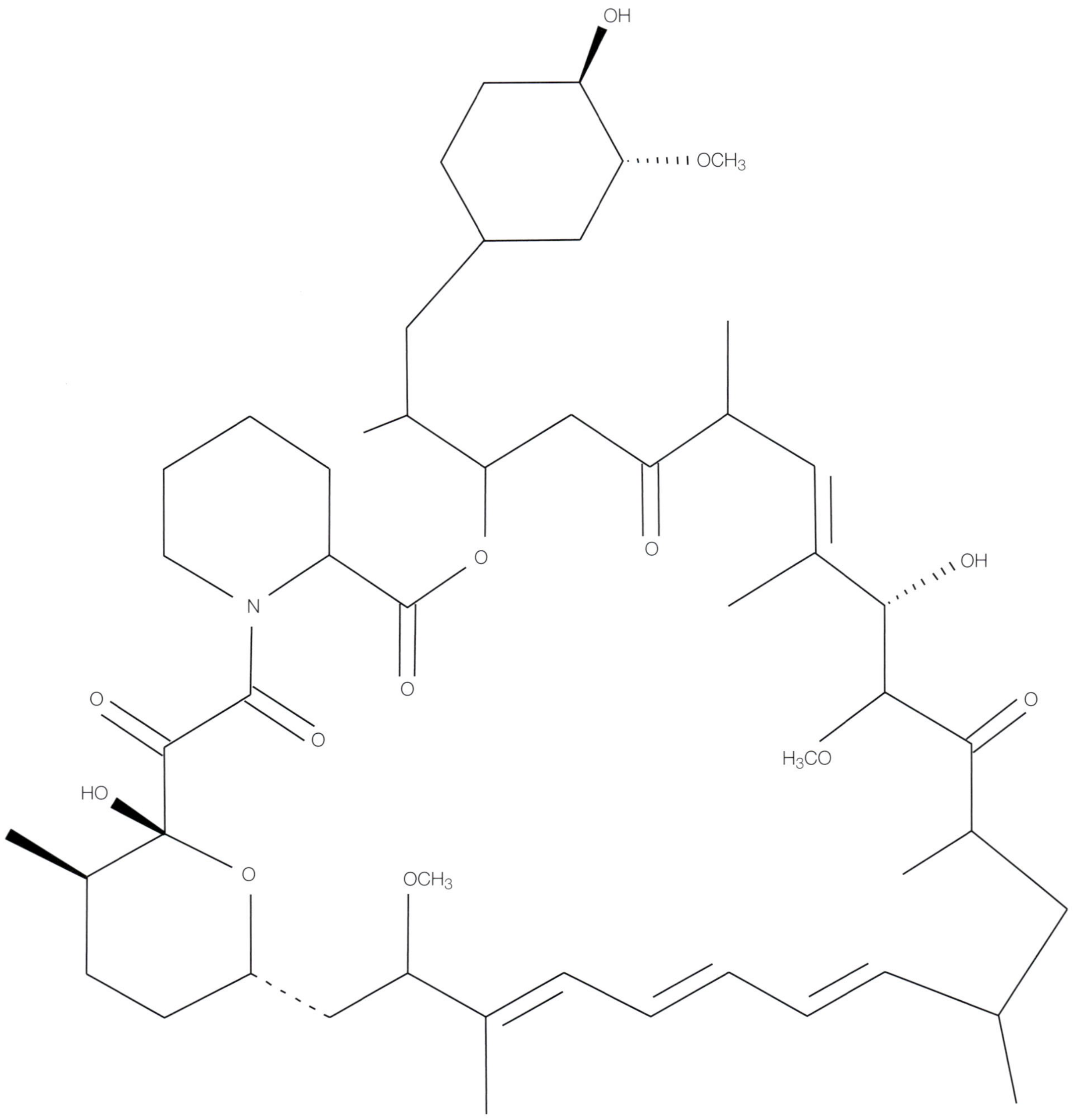

FIGURE 2-13. Chemical structure of sirolimus, mTOR inhibitor.

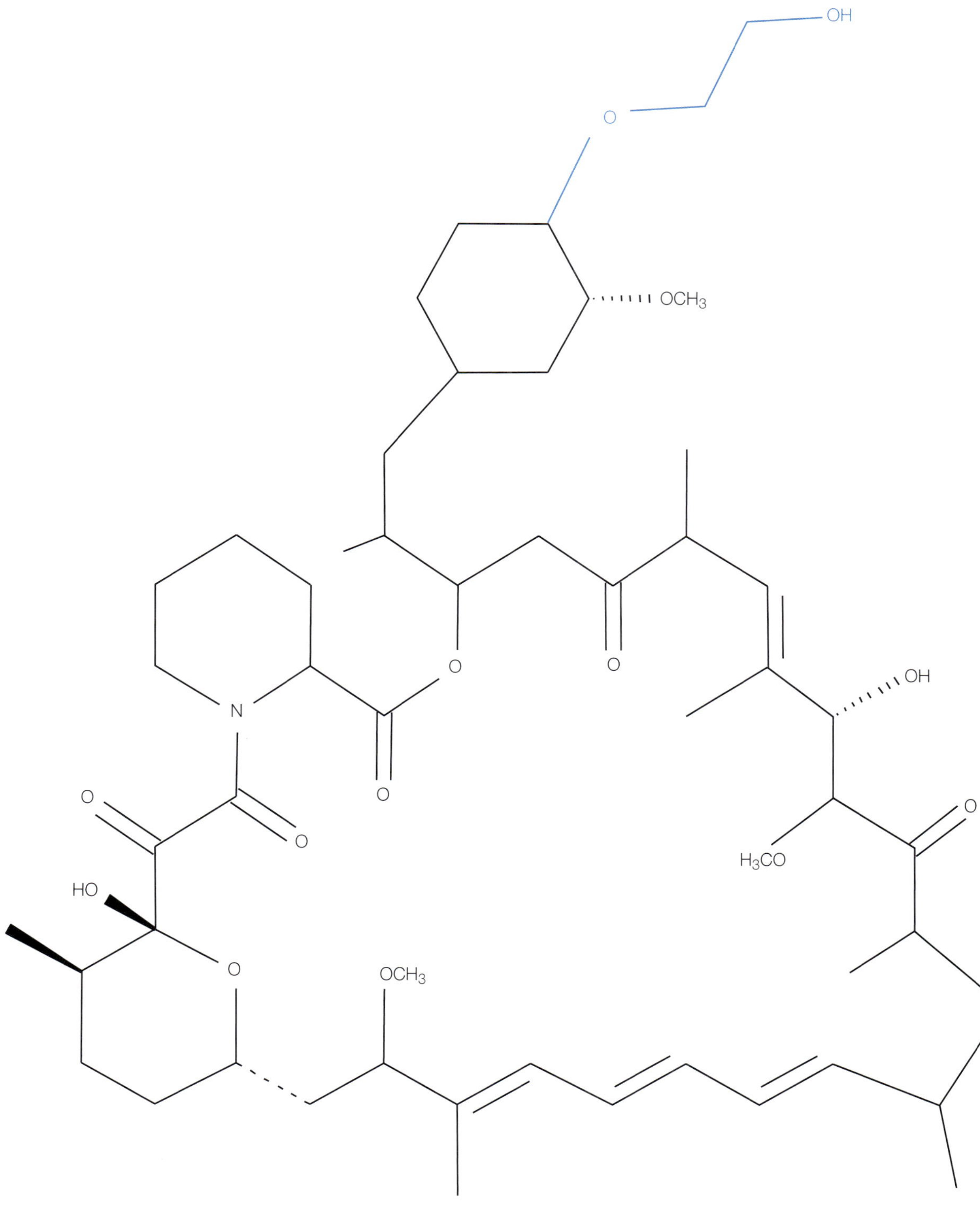

FIGURE 2-14. Chemical structure of everolimus, mTOR inhibitor.

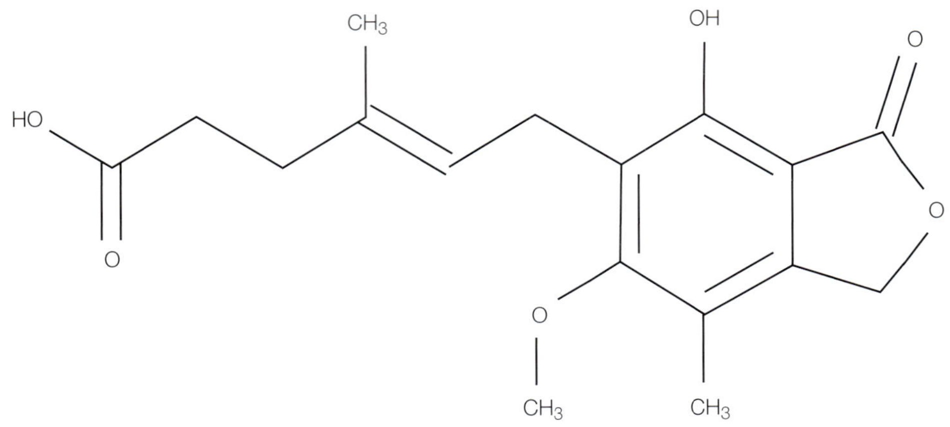

FIGURE 2-15. Chemical structure of mycophenolic acid, nucleotide synthesis inhibitor.

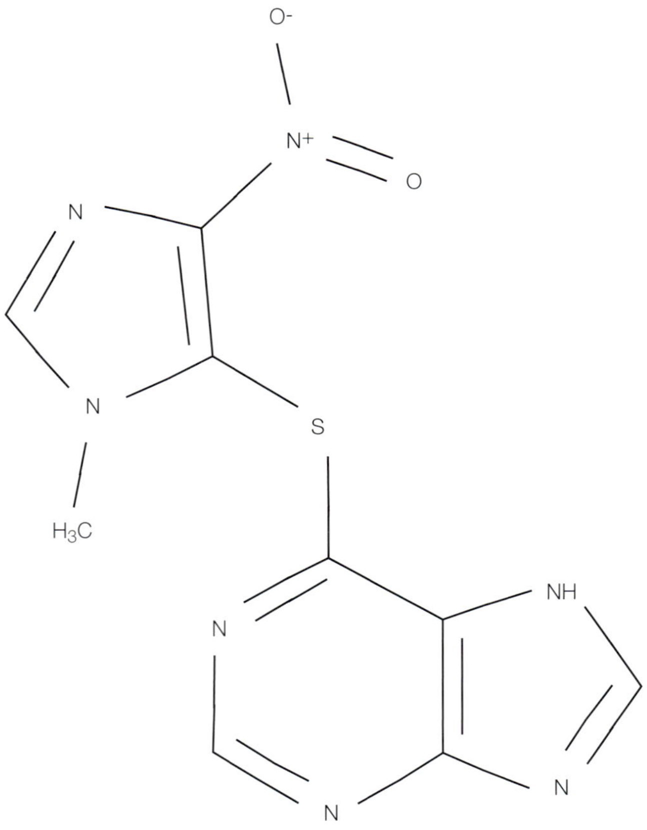

FIGURE 2-16. Chemical structure of azathioprine, nucleotide synthesis inhibitor.

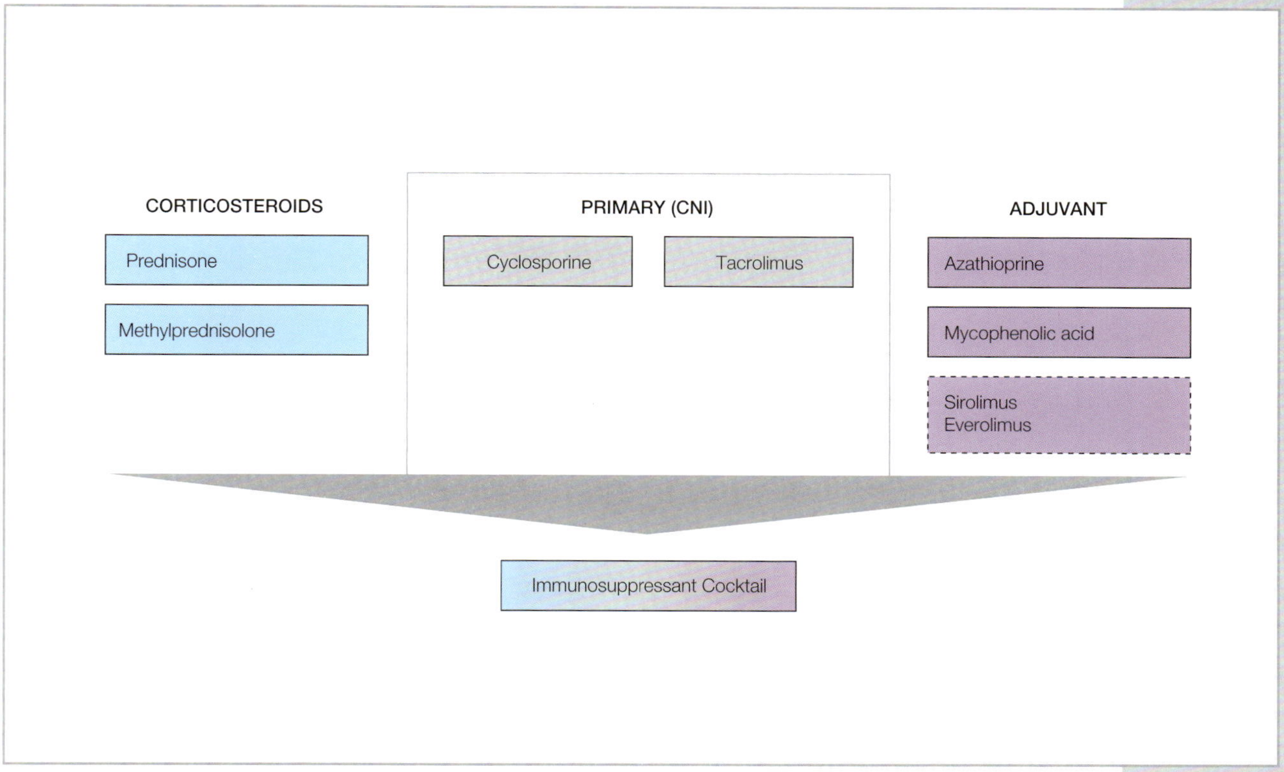

FIGURE 2-17. Immunosuppressive drug therapy.

TOXICITY OF IMMUNOSUPPRESSIVE DRUGS

Maintenance drug therapy is required throughout the life of most transplant recipients to prevent rejection of the graft. The major adverse effect of the CNIs is nephrotoxicity. As is shown in Figure 2-18, the risk of post-transplant Chronic Renal Failure (CRF) varies by the type of transplant; recipients of intestinal and liver transplants are at greatest risk. Unfortunately, there are other serious adverse effects to these medications, including neurotoxicity and an increased risk of diabetes and cardiovascular disease. The different agents all have variable adverse effect profiles as shown in Table 2-3.

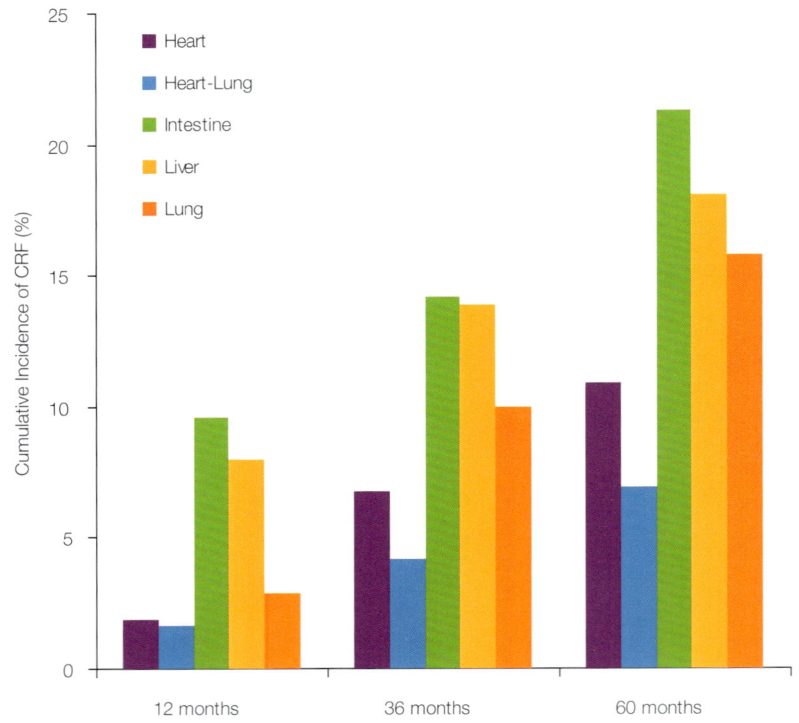

FIGURE 2-18. Cumulative incidence of chronic renal failure. Adapted from Ojo et al. (2003).

TABLE 2-3. Toxicity of Immunosuppressive Drugs

Drug	Nonimmune Toxicity
Cyclosporine	Nephrotoxicity, hypertension, neurotoxicity, gum hypertrophy, hirsutism, post-transplantation diabetes mellitus, hyperlipidemia, hemolytic-uremic syndrome
Tacrolimus	Effects similar to those of cyclosporine but with a lower incidence of hypertension, hyperlipidemia, hirsutism, and gum hyperplasia and a higher incidence of post-transplantation diabetes mellitus and neurotoxicity
Sirolimus Everolimus	Hyperlipidemia, peripheral edema, delayed wound healing, delayed graft function, mouth ulcers, pneumonitis, proteinuria
Mycophenolic acid	Gastrointestinal symptoms (mainly diarrhea), neutropenia, mild anemia
Depleting antibodies	Leukopenia, thrombocytopenia, greater risk of infection

THE PROBLEM OF GRAFT REJECTION

Over the past decade substantial progress has been made in reducing the rate of acute rejection in kidney transplant recipients. Most rejection episodes occur early after transplantation. The risk of late rejection is relatively low and often reflects non-adherence to immunosuppressive medication.

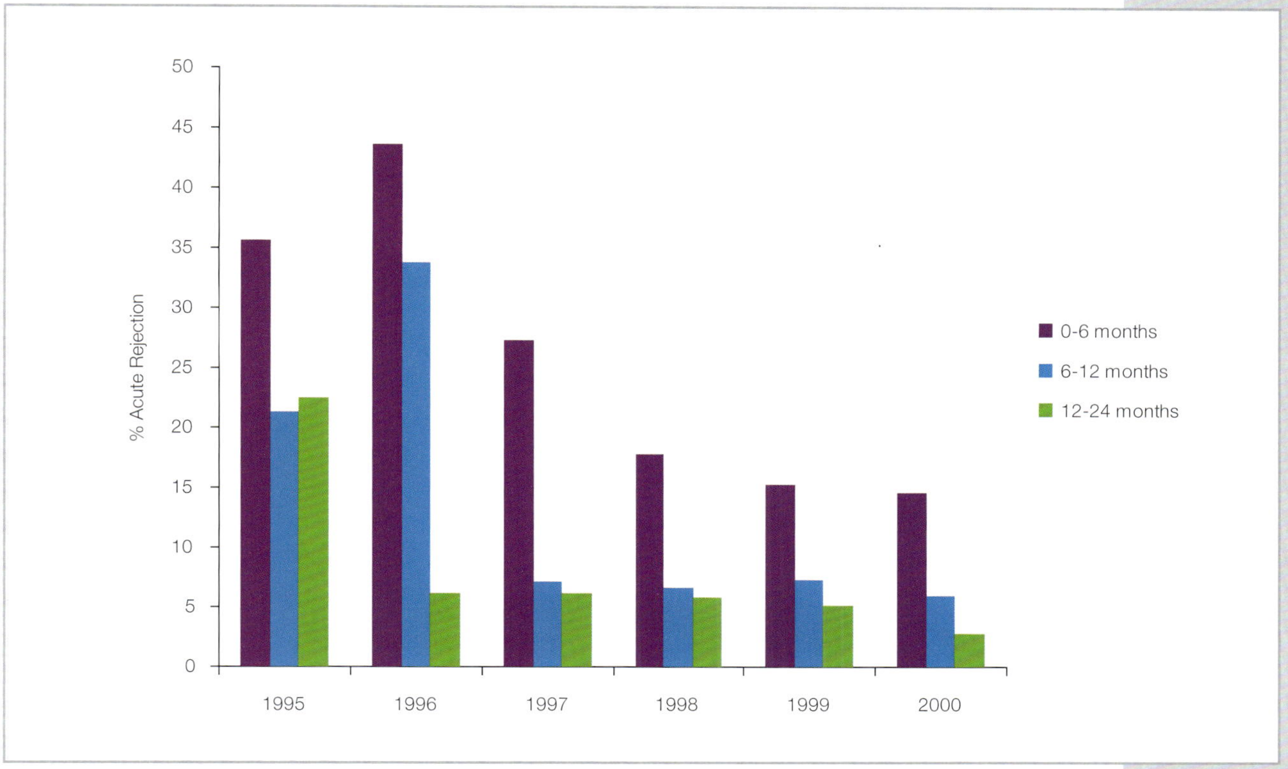

FIGURE 2-19. Incidence of early and late acute rejection episodes by era in renal allograft recipients. Adapted from Meier-Kriesche et al. (2004).

In spite of the progress in reducing the rate of acute rejection, the relative risk of renal allograft graft loss has not improved as shown below in Figure 2-20.

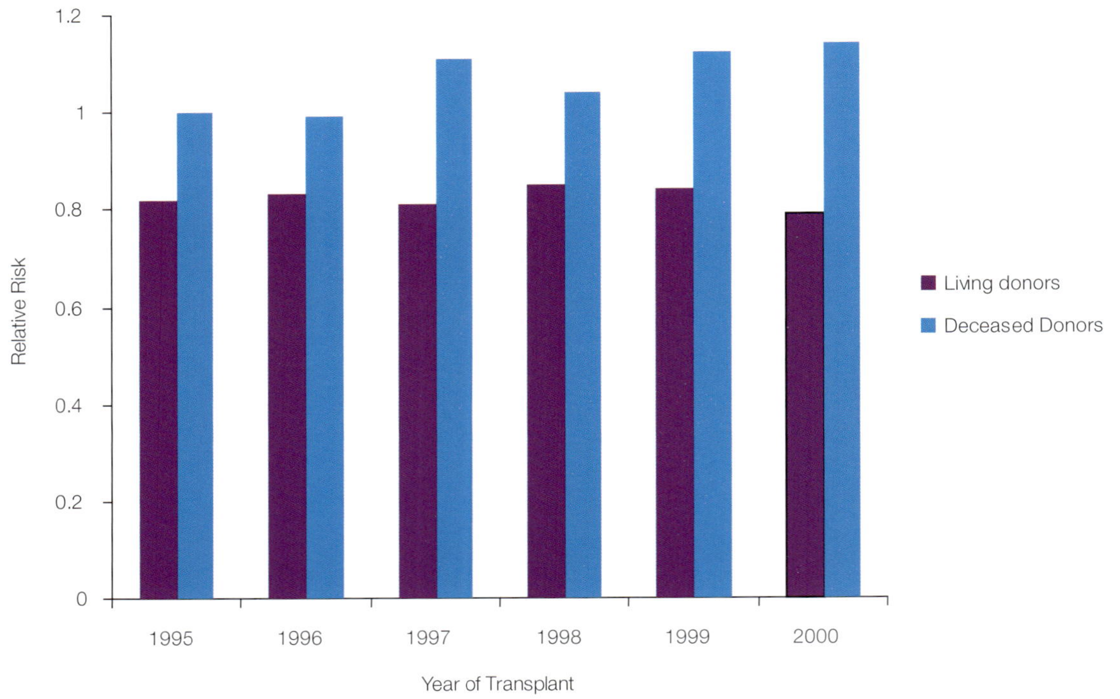

FIGURE 2-20. Relative risk for overall renal graft loss by donor type. Adapted from Meier-Kriesche et al. (2004).

As shown in the following Figures 2-21 and 2-22, the long-term survival of grafts and transplant recipients continues to be a serious problem for all organ types which has not improved much over the past 10 years.

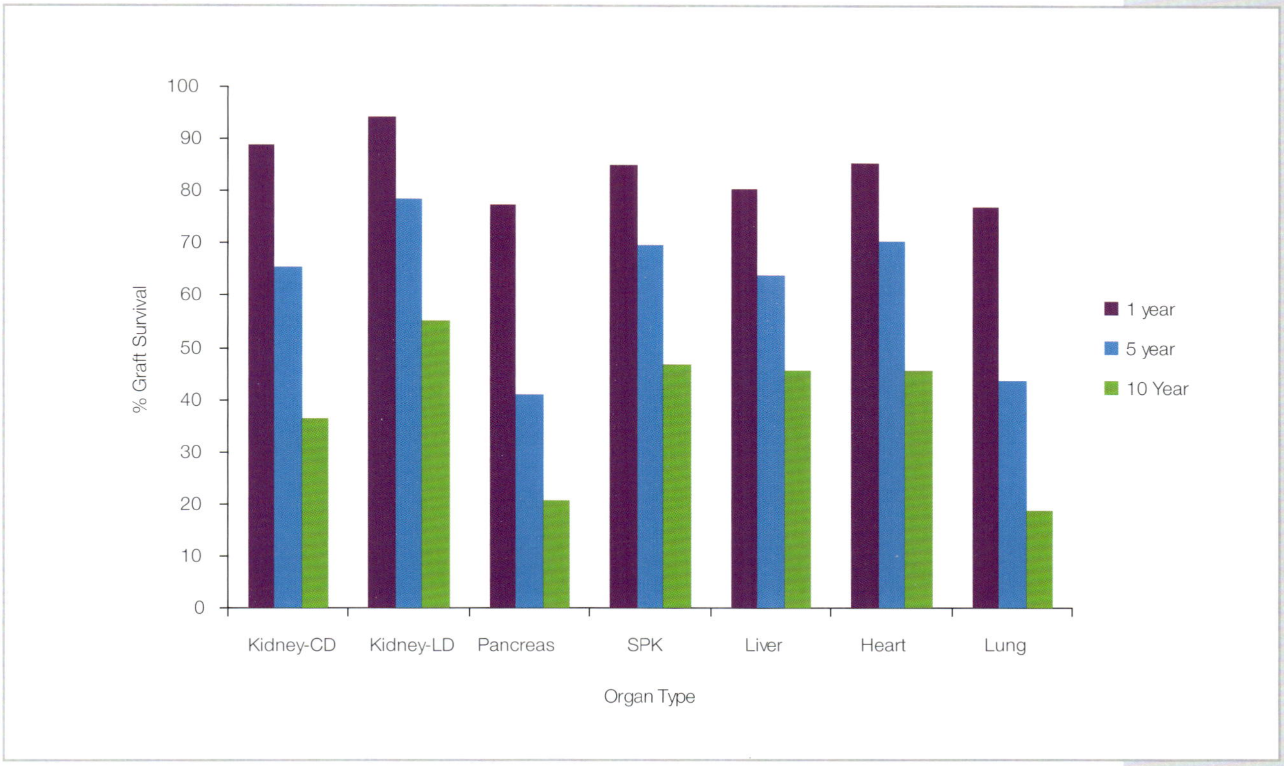

FIGURE 2-21. Graft survival by donor organ type over time. Adapted from Sayegh and Carpenter (2004).

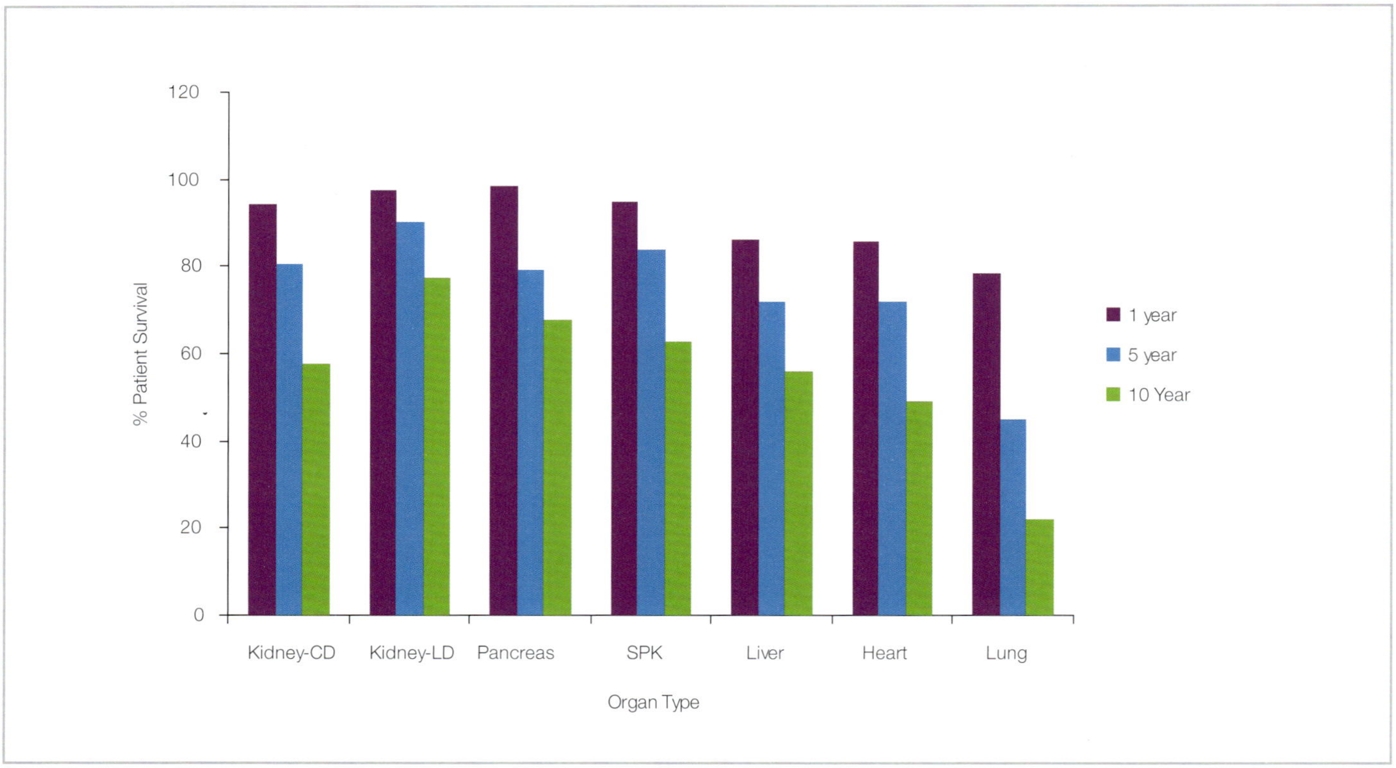

FIGURE 2-22. Patient survival by donor organ type over time. Adapted from Sayegh and Carpenter (2004).

Kidney Transplant Recipients: Chronic Allograft Nephropathy

- For kidney recipients, chronic rejection represents the most common cause of death censored graft loss. Chronic rejection is manifested by a progressive decline in renal function as measured by rising serum creatinine concentrations and proteinuria.

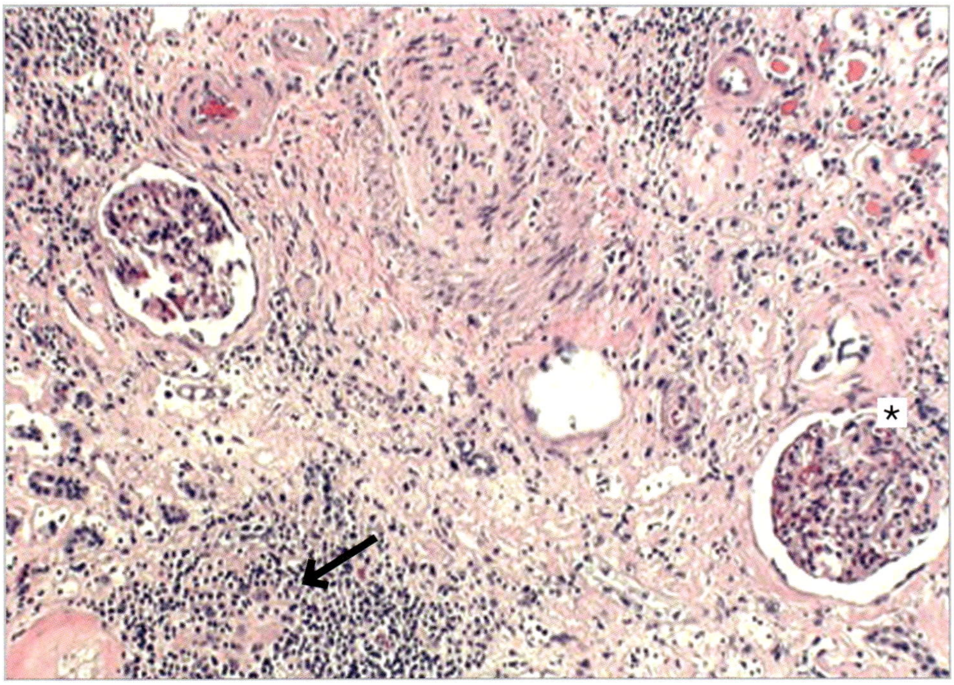

FIGURE 2-23. Chronic allograft nephropathy in a renal transplant recipient. Biopsy shows tubular atrophy and inflammation (arrow) with fibrosis and glomerular-sclerosis (asterisk).

Liver Transplant Recipients: Ductopenia and Foam Cell Arteriopathy (Jaundice)

- For liver transplant recipients, chronic rejection is an uncommon cause of graft loss. The clinical manifestation of chronic ductopenic rejection is a rising alkaline phosphatase activity followed by the onset of jaundice.

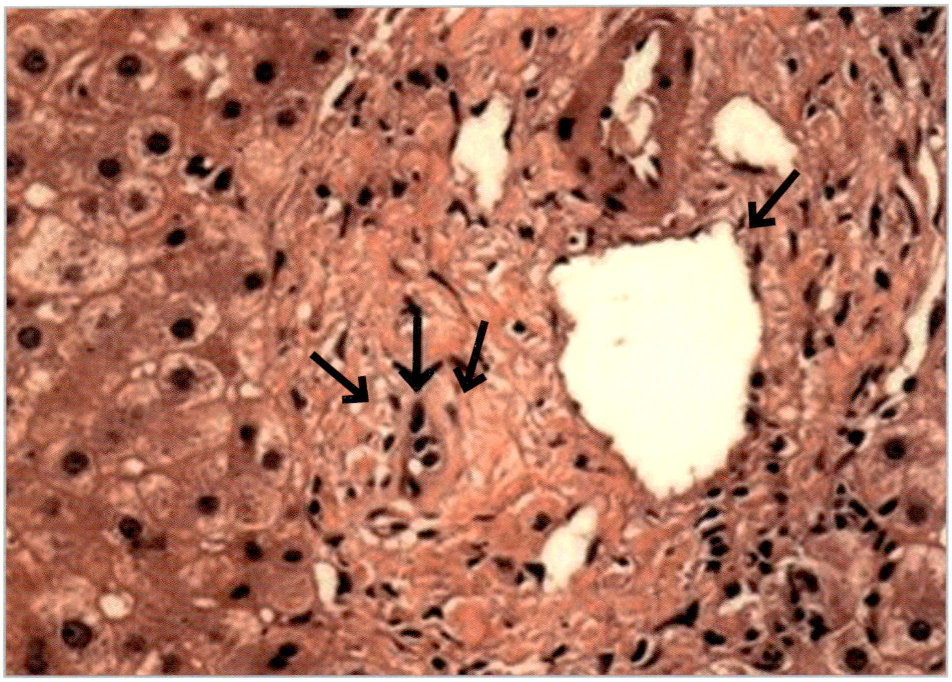

FIGURE 2-24. Evidence of ductopenic liver rejection in a transplant patient. Liver biopsy (H&E) shows portal area with normal portal vein (arrow), hepatic artery and bile ductopenia.

Heart Transplant Recipients: Post-Transplant Coronary Artery Disease (Thickening of the Arteries)

- In heart transplant recipients, the primary clinical manifestation of chronic rejection is ischemic heart disease. The diagnosis of chronic rejection or post-transplant cardiac vasculopathy can be made by endovascular ultrasonography, demonstrating neo-intimal thickening and eventually luminal obliteration.

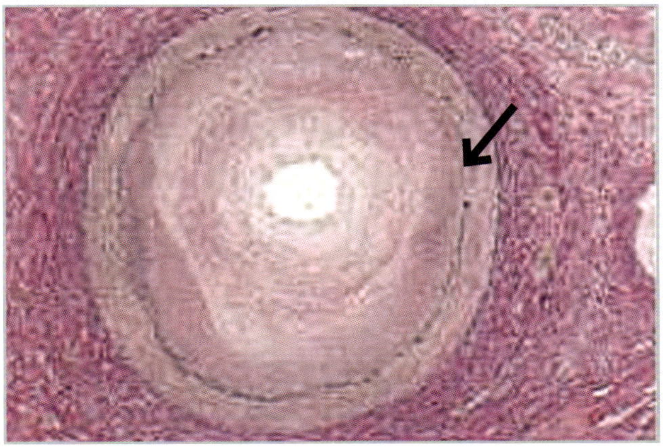

FIGURE 2-25. Ischemic heart disease in a heart transplant recipient. Biopsy from a heart transplant recipient showing marked hyperplasia with narrowing of the artery (arrow).

Lung Transplant Recipients: Bronchiolitis Obliterans (Cough)

- For lung transplant recipients, chronic rejection, or bronchiolitis obliterans, generally presents with cough, followed by a progressive decline in pulmonary function.

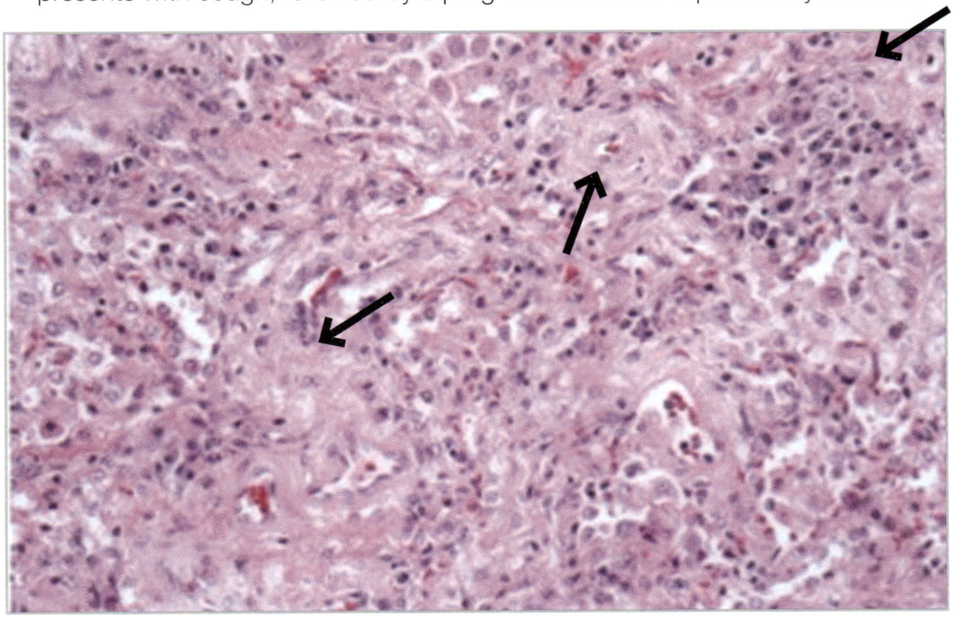

FIGURE 2-26. Bronchiolitis obliterans in a lung transplant recipient. Biopsy of a lung transplant recipient showing inflammation (arrow) and marked dilatation and loss of bronchioles.

As shown in Figure 2-27 below, the two major causes of late kidney allograft loss after the first year are chronic allograft nephropathy and death of a patient with a functioning graft. The majority of the patients who die with a functioning graft succumb to cardiovascular disease, a known risk factor for patients on immunosuppressive medication.

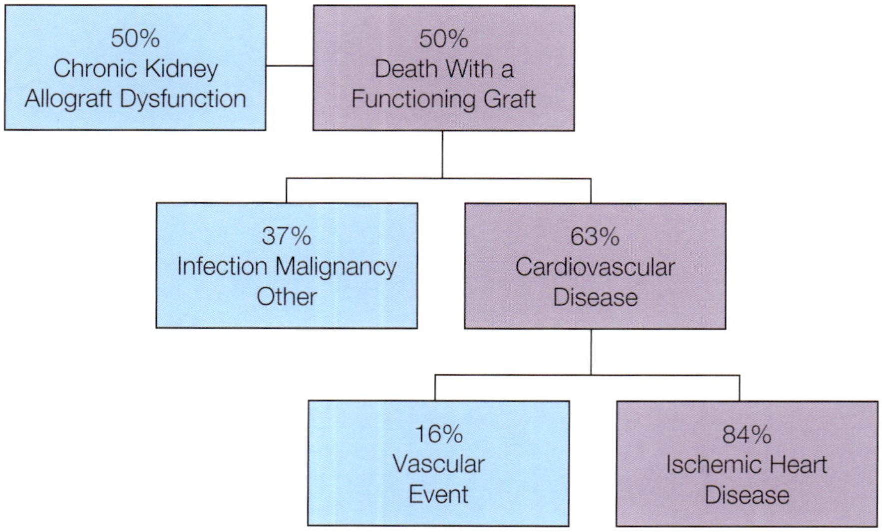

FIGURE 2-27. Causes of late kidney allograft loss. Adapted from Pascual et al. (2002) and Lindholm et al. (1995).

Maintaining the delicate balance of immunosuppression is assisted by accurate and precise measurements of the blood concentrations of the immunosuppressive drugs, but there is also a need to develop improved regimens and methods to induce graft tolerance.

DELICATE BALANCE OF IMMUNOSUPPRESSION

Too Much Immunosuppression

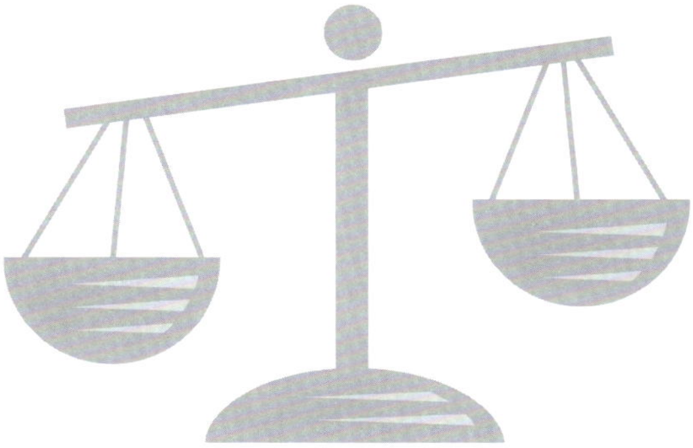

- Cardiovascular disease
  - Diabetes Mellitus
  - Hypertension
  - Hyperlipidemia
- Infection
- Nephrotoxicity
- Neoplasia
- Metabolic bone disease

Too Little Immunosuppression

- Allograft rejection

THERAPEUTIC DRUG MINIMIZATION STUDIES

Tacrolimus and cyclosporine remain staples in immunosuppression regimens, as previous attempts to remove them from the immunosuppressive cocktail were met with unacceptably high rates of acute rejection in most transplant recipients. Currently, there are no immunosuppressive regimens that can induce tolerance predictably in transplant recipients. Development of tolerence would, in theory, allow the complete removal of long-term maintenance immunosuppression. As a consequence, current studies have focused on the development of immunosuppressive regimens that minimize the use of the CNIs while maintaining adequate levels of immunosuppression and low levels of acute and chronic rejection.

ELITE-SYMPHONY STUDY

The ELITE (Efficacy Limiting Toxicity Elimination)-Symphony randomized study of Ekberg and co-workers (2007) was conducted in renal transplant recipients to assess whether a mycophenolate mofetil (MMF) based regimen would permit lower doses of CNIs, while maintaining an acceptable rate of acute rejection and a more favorable tolerability profile. Unlike previous studies, this trial utilized low dose maintenance therapy with CNIs from the day of transplantation. Patients were assigned randomly to one of four treatment groups: standard-dose cyclosporine (Normal CsA); low-dose cyclosporine (Low-CsA); low-dose tacrolimus (Low-TAC); and low-dose sirolimus (Low-SRL). The target concentrations for the four dose strategies are shown in Figure 2-28 below. The actual mean trough concentrations determined in the patients enrolled in the three low-dose regimens were biased toward the high end of the target range, whereas in the Normal CsA group the mean concentration was in line with the target. All groups received 2 g per day oral MMF.

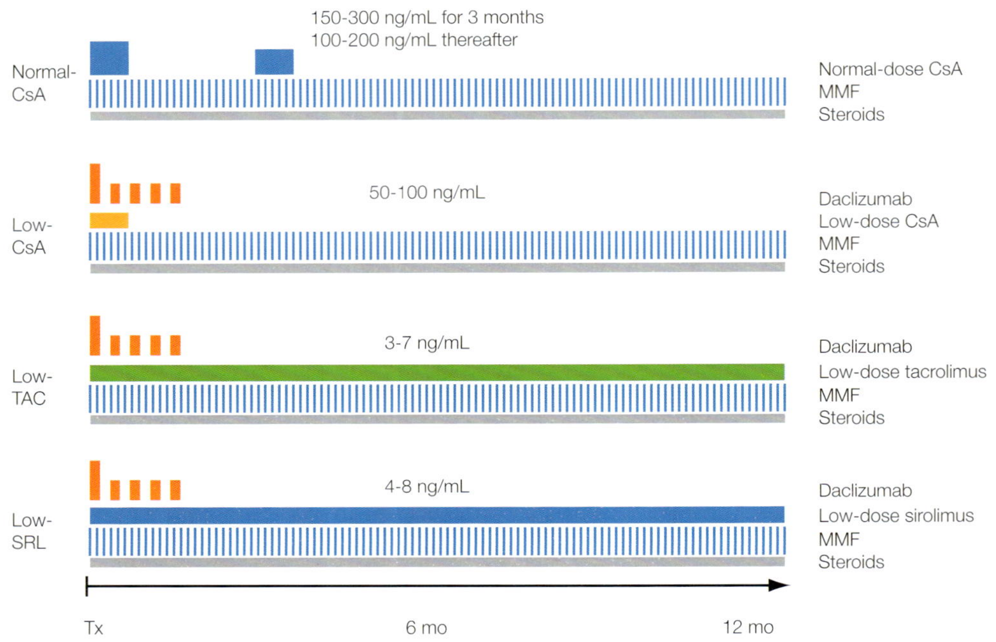

FIGURE 2-28. ELITE-Symphony Study:Drug target concentrations. Adapted from Ekberg et al. (2007).

Several end points of the ELITE-Symphony study were measured at 12 months after transplantation, including the calculated Glomerular Filtration Rate (GFR) from the serum creatinine concentrations using the Cockcroft-Gault formula, Biopsy Proven Acute Rejection (BPAR), as well as adverse events. As shown in Figure 2-29 below, the highest calculated GFR (best renal function) and the lowest incidence of BPAR were found in the low-dose tacrolimus treatment group.

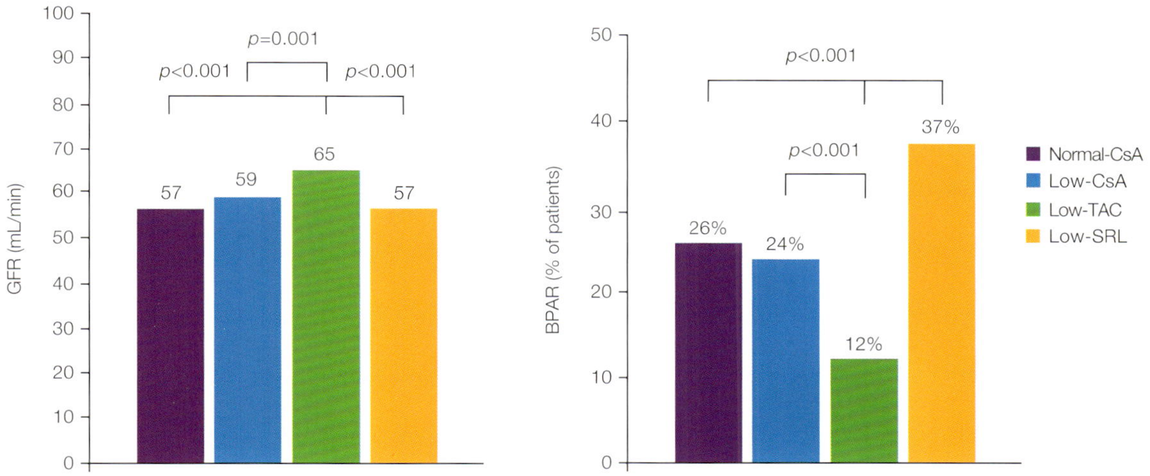

FIGURE 2-29. ELITE-Symphony Study:Calculated GFR and incidence of BPAR. Adapted from Ekberg et al. (2007).

A summary of some of the study end points and adverse events is shown in the table below. The incidence of diabetes was the highest in the low-dose tacrolimus cohort.

TABLE 2-4. ELITE-Symphony Study: Selected End Points and Adverse Events.

End Points and Adverse Events	Standard Dose Cyclosporine (N=390)	Low Dose Cyclosporine (N=401)	Low Dose Tacrolimus (N=401)	Low Dose Sirolimus (N=399)	P Value
Mean calculated GFR-ml/min	57.1 ± 25.1	59.4 ± 25.1	65.4 ± 27.1	56.7 ± 26.9	<0.001
P Value for Comparison w/ Tacrolimus	<0.001	0.001	Reference	<0.001	
Allograft Survival	91.9%	94.3%	96.4%	91.7%	0.02
P Value for Comparison w/ Tacrolimus	0.007	0.18	Reference	0.007	
Hypertension	14.3%	11.5%	12.9%	11.8%	
Diabetes mellitus	6.0%	4.2%	8.4%	6.6%	
Hyperlipidemia	14.8%	12.5%	9.9%	15.8%	
Increased blood creatinine concentration	7.8%	6.9%	8.2%	7.9%	

Adapted from Ekberg et al. (2007).

The main conclusion of the ELITE-Symphony study was that an immunosuppressive regimen consisting of daclizumab induction, MMF, low dose tacrolimus and corticosteroids in renal transplant recipients may lead to fewer adverse effects, while maintaining good renal function, low acute rejection rates, and improved patient survival and quality of life.

SIROLIMUS-BASED, CNI SPARING THERAPY

The requirement for CNI agents in immunosuppression regimens to prevent acute rejection has led investigators to investigate alternative therapies that can safely reduce the levels of these agents during long-term maintenance therapy. Recently, Conti and co-workers (2008) reported on their six year experience using a sirolimus-based, CNI sparing, dose regimen in a cohort of 50 consecutive primary renal transplant recipients. The patients were treated initially with a triple drug regimen consisting of prednisone, sirolimus targeted to a 24 hour trough concentration of 8-12 ng/mL, and tacrolimus targeted to a 12 hour trough concentration of 8-12 ng/mL. After 90 days the tacrolimus dosing was decreased by 50% with subsequent dosing targeted to achieve a 12 hour trough blood concentration of 2-3 ng/mL.

The mean tacrolimus concentrations, patient and graft survival, and renal function as a function of time post-transplant are shown in Figures 2-30, 2-31, and 2-32, respectively. It should be noted that the mean maintenance tacrolimus concentrations in this study were half. i.e. <3 ng/mL versus a mean concentration closer to 7 ng/mL in the ELITE-Symphony study. The incidence of early acute rejection (< 3 months) was only 10% and no late rejection episodes occurred. The authors concluded that sirolimus may allow for the reduction of maintenance CNI dosing.

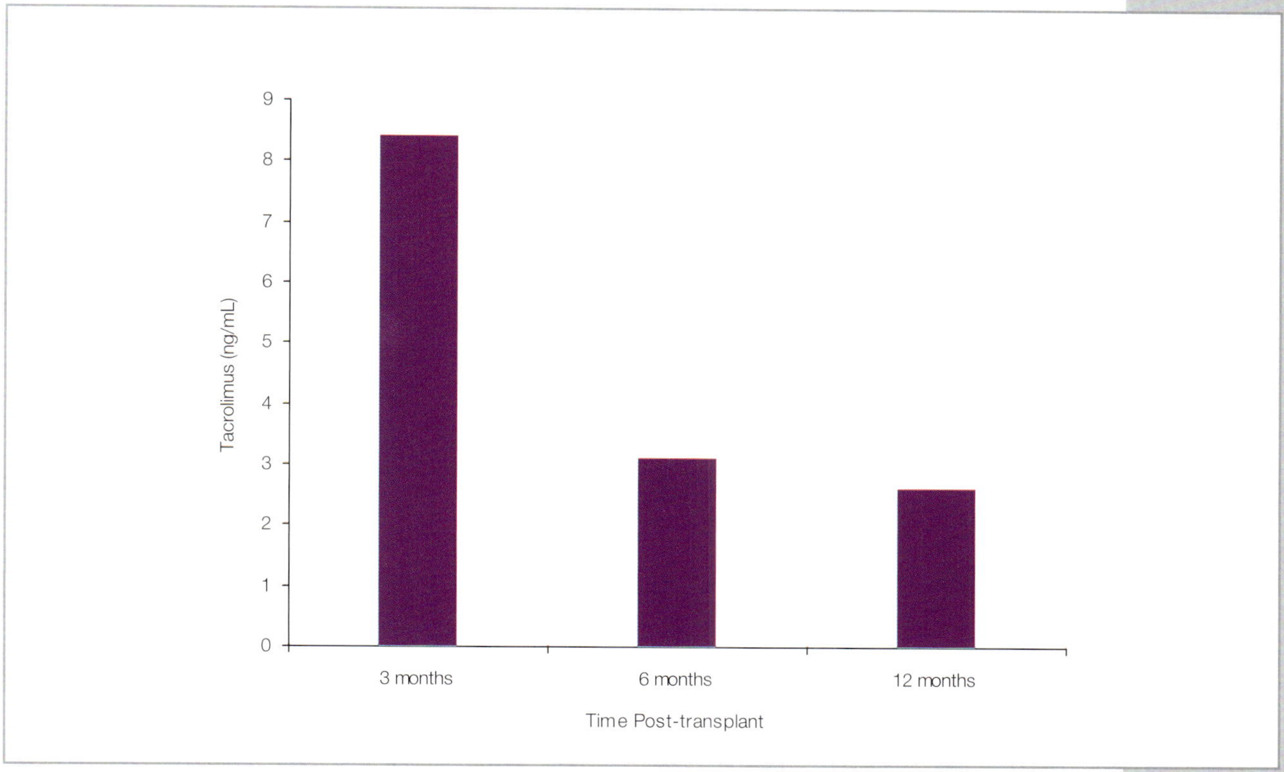

FIGURE 2-30. Mean tacrolimus blood concentrations in patients undergoing sirolimus-based CNI sparing therapy. Adapted from Conti et al. (2008).

The optimization of immunosuppressive therapy and improvement of quality of life in solid organ transplant recipients continues to be an active area of research. The studies of Ekberg et al. (2007) and Conti et al. (2008) have demonstrated that lower trough blood concentrations of tacrolimus can be achieved in renal allograft recipients while maintaining an acceptable rate of acute rejection. The long-term benefit of reduced tacrolimus concentrations in these patients remains to be determined. As researchers continue to explore novel regimens employing lower concentrations of CNIs, improved therapeutic drug monitoring methods will be necessary to accurately and precisely measure these low blood concentrations.

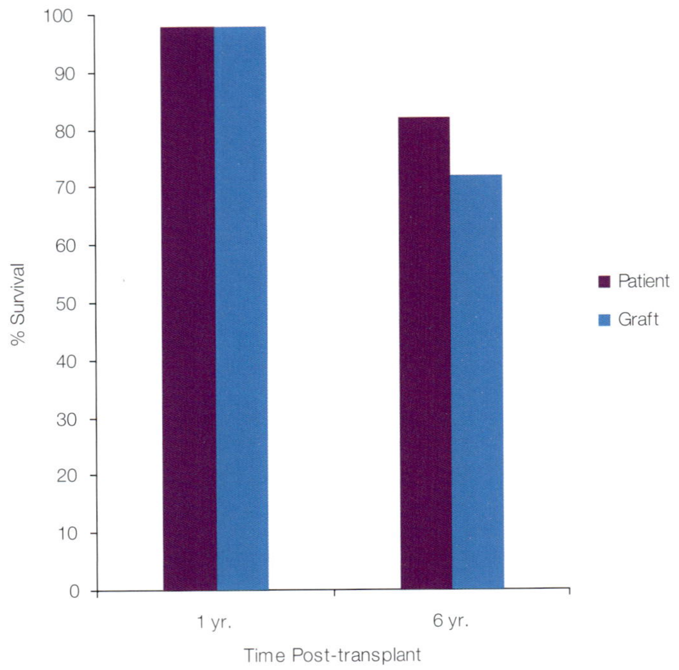

FIGURE 2-31. Survival in patients undergoing sirolimus-based CNI sparing therapy. Adapted from Conti et al. (2008).

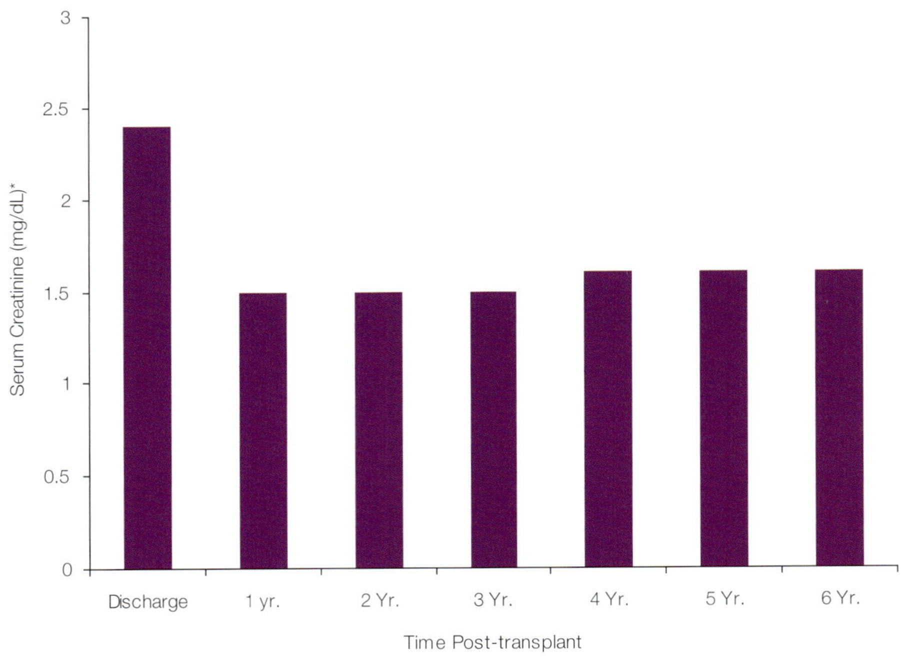

*1 mg/dL = 88.4 µmol/L

FIGURE 2-32. Renal function in patients undergoing sirolimus-based CNI sparing therapy. Adapted from Conti et al. (2008).

BIBLIOGRAPHY FOR CHAPTER 2

Halloran PF. Immunosuppressive drugs for kidney transplantation. N Engl J Med. 2004;351:2715-29.

Ojo AO, Held PJ, Port FK, Wolfe RA, Leichtman AB, Young EW, Arndorfer J, Christensen L, Merion RM. Chronic renal failure after transplantation of a nonrenal organ. N Engl J Med. 2003;349:931-40.

Meier-Kreische HU, Schold JD, Srinivas TR, Kaplan B. Lack of improvement in renal allograft survival despite a marked decrease in acute rejection rates over the most recent era. Am J Transplant. 2004; 4:378-83.

Sayegh MH, Carpenter CB. Transplantation 50 years later-progress, challenges, and promises. N Engl J Med. 2004;351:2761-6.

Pascual M, Theruvath T, Kawai T et al. Strategies to improve long-term outcomes after renal transplantation. N Engl J Med. 2002;346:580-90.

Lindholm A, Albrechtsen D, Frodin L et al. Ischemic heart disease-major cause of death and graft loss after renal transplantation in scandinavia. Transplant. 1995;60:451-6.

Ekberg E, Tedesco-Silva H, Demirbas A et al. Reduced exposure to calcineurin inhibitors in renal transplantation. N Engl J Med. 2007;357:2562-75.

Conti DJ, Petrov R, Elbalhoul O, Gallichio M. Sirolimus-based, calcineurin-inhibitor sparing immunotherapy, long-term (6-year) results. Transplant Immunol. 2008;20:12-13.

Meier-Kriesche HU, Li S, Gruessner RWG et al. Immunosuppression:Evolution in practice and trends, 1994-2004. Am J Transplant. 2006;6:1111-31.

03 THERAPEUTIC DRUG MONITORING OF IMMUNOSUPPRESSIVE DRUGS

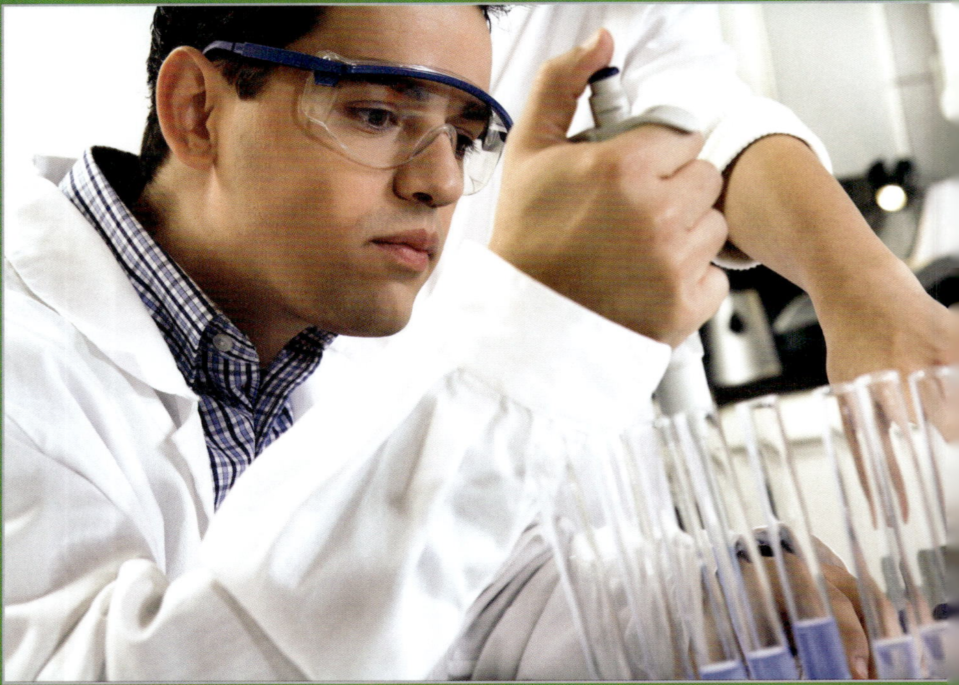

CHAPTER 3 CONTENTS

03 THERAPEUTIC DRUG MONITORING OF IMMUNOSUPPRESSIVE DRUGS

INTRODUCTION TO TDM

Therapeutic Drug Monitoring (TDM) of Immunosuppressive Drugs

TDM uses repeated measurements of a drug in plasma or whole blood as a guide to drug dosing. Clinicians find these measurements of value when:

- Drugs exert their therapeutic effects over a narrow range of drug concentrations, sometimes called the therapeutic range.
- Symptoms and signs of drug toxicity are not specific to the drug, and may be difficult to distinguish from under dosage.
- The concentration of a drug in blood is a better guide to its efficacy than knowledge of the dose prescribed.
- Drugs are prescribed in combination with other drugs that can raise or lower the concentration of the drug of interest. These drug interactions (see p. 70) can be identified, and therapy adjusted accordingly, using TDM.
- Poor compliance (adherence) with the prescribed dose is suspected.

Drugs that need to be monitored:

- Critical Dose Drugs, i.e. those drugs for which small changes in dose can result in changes in drug exposure that result in drug toxicity or loss of efficacy.
- Drugs with a clinical effect that is difficult to quantify.
- When the relationship between dose and blood concentration is unpredictable.
- When the drug is given over a prolonged period of time.

The underlying rationale for TDM is illustrated in Figure 3-1. A clear relationship between drug concentrations and both efficacy and toxicity is evident. TDM becomes of value as the two concentration curves become closer, i.e. the ratio between therapy and toxicity (the therapeutic index) becomes smaller.

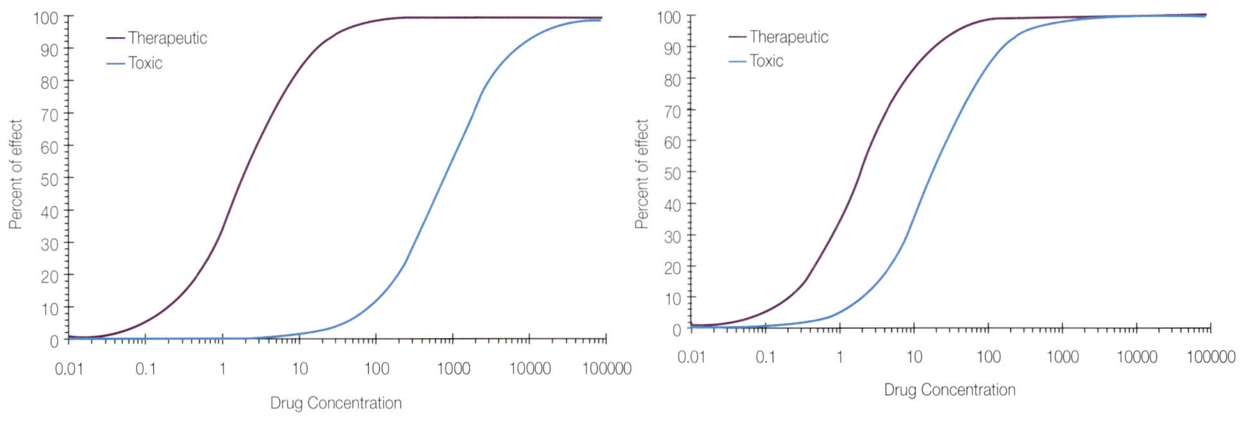

FIGURE 3-1. Relationship between drug concentration, efficacy and toxicity.

03 THERAPEUTIC DRUG MONITORING OF IMMUNOSUPPRESSIVE DRUGS

IMMUNOSUPPRESSIVE DRUG MONITORING

Since their introduction, there has been interest in the measurement of cyclosporine, tacrolimus, sirolimus and everolimus in blood as a guide to dose adjustment. In some countries, the measurement of sirolimus and everolimus is actually a regulatory requirement.

For the calcineurin inhibitors, cyclosporine and tacrolimus, the introduction of TDM was a rather *ad hoc* development. The results have been very dependent on the analytical method used and the choice of sample matrix. Early attempts at TDM for these drugs was based on the use of plasma or serum, until it was established that both cyclosporine and tacrolimus tended to concentrate in red cells, resulting in higher blood concentrations than plasma or serum concentrations. As a result, consensus documents on TDM for these drugs recommended that the measurements should be made in a whole blood sample. Sirolimus and everolimus, both introduced at a later date, are also concentrated in red cells, so TDM of these drugs is also performed using a whole blood sample.

For all of these drugs there are no randomized controlled studies comparing outcomes if dosing is based on TDM, rather than fixed dose adjusted on the basis of symptoms or signs alone. For sirolimus and everolimus several clinical studies based on TDM were performed during their early use in patients. These studies established a clear relationship between blood concentration and either efficacy or toxicity.

The interest in dosing these drugs based on blood concentration measurements, rather than on the basis of fixed doses, stems from the poor correlation between dose and exposure to the drug. This is illustrated in Figure 3-2, which shows blood concentration-time curves in a group of volunteer subjects receiving the same dose of sirolimus. It is clear that these subjects were exposed to very different amounts of the drug, as assessed by area under the concentration-time curve (AUC) or by the final pre-dose concentration at 24 hours after dosing. When the drug is given to transplant patients an even wider dispersion of results can be anticipated, because of intercurrent illness and the effects of other drug therapy. A clinician knowing only the dose prescribed really has no idea of the patient's actual exposure to the drug.

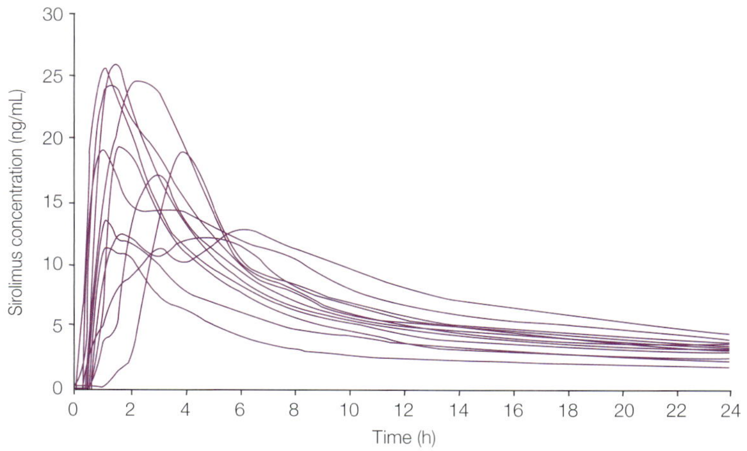

FIGURE 3-2. Sirolimus concentrations in whole blood samples collected from 12 healthy volunteers given a single dose of 6mg sirolimus. There is a wide dispersion of results, in terms of AUC, time to maximum concentration t_{max}, maximum concentration C_{max} and the concentration at the end of the dosing interval. Data - Analytical Unit, St George's – University of London, unpublished.

The exception among the commonly used immunosuppressive drugs is mycophenolic acid (MPA). This drug is usually given in combination with at least one of the above drugs, and has tended to be dosed on the basis of a fixed dose regimen. Recently, there have been two clinical trials in which patients were either dosed on the basis of TDM or by fixed doses. The results were equivocal, one study showing an advantage to TDM, the other no advantage.

So, with the above points in mind, is there a good case for the measurement of immunosuppressive drugs?

SPECIFIC PROBLEMS RELATED TO IMMUNOSUPPRESSIVE DRUGS

Cyclosporine, tacrolimus, sirolimus and everolimus are generally considered to be Critical Dose Drugs. There are some aspects of these drugs which make them prime candidates for TDM.

- Multiple drug therapy is common in the management of patients who have received an organ transplant. Not only immunosuppressive drugs have to be considered. Other classes of drugs, such as antibiotics, lipid lowering therapy and anti-hypertensives have the potential to produce pharmacokinetic drug interactions (altering one or more drug concentration).
- Patients are probably going to receive immunosuppressive drugs for the rest of their lives, so remembering to take them, or deliberately failing to take them, is a distinct possibility.
- All these drugs have serious adverse effects, which can appear at doses well within the normal dose range. Anything that can help the clinician to tailor the dose before these effects are seen is of value.
- Some of the adverse effects, such as a decline in kidney function, are also the effects that could result from underdosing, resulting in graft rejection. Distinguishing between these two clinical effects is not always easy, and drug measurements can help in the differential diagnosis.

Measurement of cyclosporine, tacrolimus, sirolimus and everolimus are made using whole blood rather than plasma or serum as the sample matrix for the reason noted above. The low concentrations found in plasma or serum during normal therapy would be challenging for any of the routine analytical techniques in use today.

MPA is not usually considered to be a Critical Dose Drug, but it is well known that for any given dose there is a wide between-subject variation in exposure, as measured by AUC, and that exposure is related to the clinical effects of the drug. Interpretation of MPA concentrations is complicated by the fact that the drug is almost always given in combination with another immunosuppressive drug, so the body's immune response is being influenced by more than one drug. Therefore, there is little point in measuring MPA without ensuring that concentrations of cyclosporine or tacrolimus are also adequate.

Measurements of MPA are made in plasma or serum; the drug is not distributed into red blood cells. Results are not valid if the sample has been hemolyzed. The data used for the interpretation of MPA concentrations are mostly based on pharmacokinetic findings following the use of the mycophenolate mofetil formulation (CellCept®). There is also an enteric coated formulation (Myfortic®). This formulation is not absorbed until after it has passed through the stomach, so the time to maximum concentration is delayed compared with mycophenolate mofetil. In some instances, absorption can be slowed for some hours because of delayed gastric emptying. As a result:

- The kinetics of the two formulations vary so widely that the algorithms used to calculate AUC, derived using mycophenolate mofetil, cannot be used if the patient is taking the enteric coated formulation.
- Because the peak concentration can be some hours after dosing, pre-dose (trough) concentrations may be higher when the enteric formulation is used.

Always check which MPA formulation the patient is taking.

PHARMACOKINETICS

The science of pharmacokinetics studies the effect the body has on a drug, that is, how the drug is absorbed by the body, the distribution of the drug throughout the body, metabolism of the drug, and its excretion. Most of the immunosuppressive drugs display a high volume of distribution (Vd) > 1 L/kg, are largely bound to plasma proteins (albumin, α1 glycoprotein acid, lipoproteins) and to erythrocytes (except MPA, which remains in the plasma fraction). Pharmacokinetic parameters for immunosuppressive drugs are listed in Table 3-1.

Calcineurin inhibitors (cyclosporine and tacrolimus) and mTOR inhibitors (sirolimus and everolimus) are extensively oxidized by the cytochrome CYP3A subfamily of enzymes. Most of these metabolites are inactive. A large number of hydroxylated and O- or N-demethylated metabolites have been identified: > 30 for cyclosporine; > 9 for tacrolimus; > 11 for everolimus; and > 13 metabolites for sirolimus. Mycophenolate mofetil, as a prodrug, is rapidly de-esterified to form MPA. MPA is converted to the 7-O-MPA-β-glucuronide (MPAG), the primary (inactive) metabolite, via different isoforms of uridine diphosphate glucuronosyltransferase (UGT). Three additional MPA metabolites, M-1 (phenolic 7-OH glucoside conjugate), M-2 (acyl glucuronide conjugate or Ac-MPAG, displaying some residual activity), and M-3 (6-O-desmethyl-MPA) have been identified. Metabolites for immunosuppressive drugs are listed in Table 3-2.

The age of the patient is an important factor affecting drug disposition. Pediatric patients clear immunosuppressive drugs from the blood more rapidly than adults. Children <5 years, or between 5-12 years of age, will need a higher tacrolimus dose as compared to adults, 2.7 or 1.9 fold, respectively.

03 THERAPEUTIC DRUG MONITORING OF IMMUNOSUPPRESSIVE DRUGS

TABLE 3-1. Pharmacokinetic Parameters

	Cyclosporine	Tacrolimus	Sirolimus	Everolimus	MMF (MPA)	EC-MPS (MPA)
F (%)	15-40	25 (5-93)	10-14	16	80.7-94	72
Vd/F (L/kg)	1.0-1.6	0.85-1.67	5.6-16.7	1.5	3.8-5.3	
Cl/F (L/h/kg)	0.12-0.7	0.04-0.14	0.09-0.42	0.12	14.1-34.9 L/h (CsA) 11.9-25.4 L/h (Tac)	
$t_{1/2}$ (h)	6-20.5	3.5-40.5	46.1-78.5	18-35	9-17	9-17
Fu (%)	3	1	8	5-10	1-3	1-3
t_{max} (h)	1-4	0.5-1	3.1±2.4	1.5-2	1-2 4-12 (2nd peak)	1.5-2.75
Ratio blood/plasma	3-5	15 (4-114)	36.5		NA plasma	NA plasma

F: oral bioavailability
Vd/F : apparent volume of distribution
Cl/F: apparent clearance
$t_{1/2}$: elimination half-life
t_{max}: time to peak concentration
Fu: free fraction

MMF: Mycophenolate Mofetil (CellCept) formulation of MPA
EC-MPS: Enteric Coated Mycophenolate Sodium (Myfortic) formulation of MPA.

TABLE 3-2. Metabolites of Immunosuppressive Drugs

Cyclosporine metabolites	Activity %	Metabolite* abundance at C_0%
AM 1 1-β-hydroxyl	10-20	80-150
AM 9 9-γ-hydroxyl	5-10	50-75
AM 4N 4 N-demethyl	3-5	5-25

Tacrolimus metabolites	Activity %	Metabolite* abundance at C_0%
M I 13-O demethyl	6.4	6
M II 31-O demethyl	100	15
M III 15-O-demethyl	0	6
M IV 12-O-hydroxyl	3.5	NR
M V 15,31-O-didemethyl	0	NR

Sirolimus metabolites	Activity %	Metabolite* abundance at C_0%
39-O-demethyl	10	5
12-hydroxyl	7	11
46-hydroxyl	NR	7
24-hydroxyl	NR	9.8
16-O-demethyl	NR	8.6

Everolimus metabolites	Activity %	Metabolite* abundance at C_0%
46-hydroxyl	NR	44.1
24-hydroxyl	NR	7.7
25-hydroxyl	NR	14.4
demethyl	NR	<1

* Metabolite abundance relative to parent drug concentration at the trough concentration, expressed in percentage NR=Not Reported.

PHARMACOKINETICS AND DRUG INTERACTIONS

Once the drug passes through the gut wall, it undergoes some intestinal first-pass effect (oxidized by the CYP3A4 or CYP3A5 present in the enterocytes) and is a substrate of a transporter protein, such as P-glycoprotein (P-gp). These processes limit the amount of drug reaching the portal vein and the liver. The fraction of the immunosuppressive drug that reaches the liver undergoes hepatic first-pass effect. A fraction of the drug reaching the liver is metabolized during this first-pass effect. Therefore, the oral bioavailability (F) corresponds to the final fraction of the drug which reaches the systemic circulation and is available to target sites for pharmacological activity as shown in Figure 3-3.

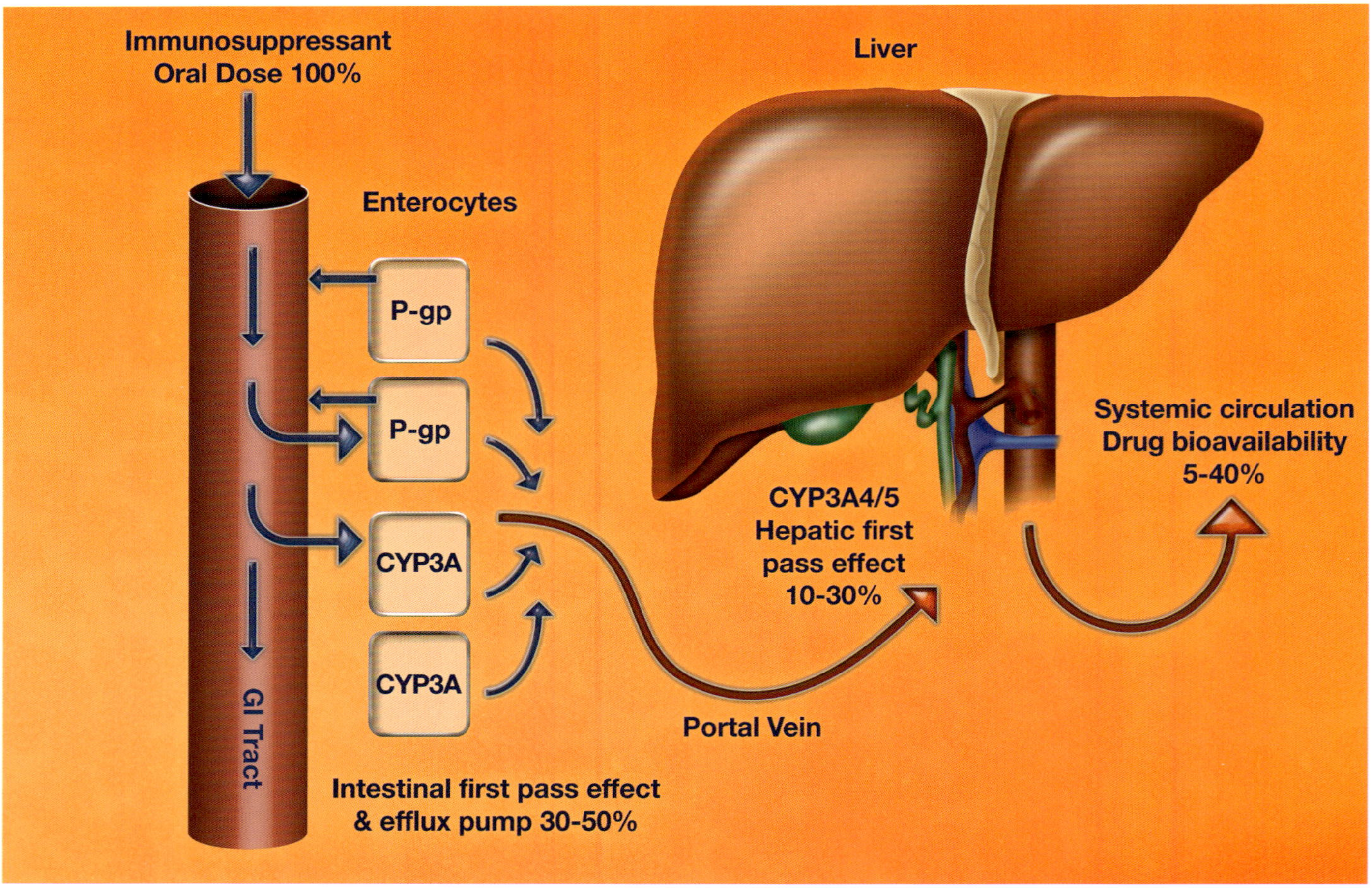

FIGURE 3-3. Drug metabolism and oral bioavailability.

The oral bioavailability of immunosuppressive drugs is highly variable, and may depend on a number of factors such as:

- Liver and GI tract function (liver dysfunction, bile flow, diarrhea, GI surgery, enzyme maturation or expression).
- Food and diet.
- Time (morning versus evening) and time post-transplantation (F increases over the first few months).
- Drug interactions.
- Transporter protein expression.

03 THERAPEUTIC DRUG MONITORING OF IMMUNOSUPPRESSIVE DRUGS

The frequency of drug-drug interactions is high in most solid organ transplant recipients because of polypharmacy. These interactions (mostly induction or inhibition) involve, predominantly, the cytochrome P450 (CYP) enzymes and the P-gp, occurring either at the hepatic or intestinal levels.

Other mechanisms of drug interactions have been described. Mycophenolic acid undergoes some enterohepatic recirculation, contributing significantly to its bioavailability. For the same dose, MPA concentrations are lower in transplant recipients receiving mycophenolate mofetil (MMF) and cyclosporine compared with those receiving MMF with tacrolimus. Cyclosporine inhibits MPA glucuronide (MPAG) excretion into bile, and, consequently, decreases enterohepatic recirculation of MPA. Tables 3-3 and 3-4 (tacrolimus), 3-5 (cyclosporine), 3-6 (sirolimus), and 3-7 (everolimus) describe the effects other drugs and agents have on immunosuppressive drug concentrations in blood.

TABLE 3-3. Drugs That May Increase Tacrolimus Blood Concentration

Calcium Channel Blockers	Antifungal Agents	Macrolide Antibiotics
diltiazem	clotrimazole	clarithromycin
nicardipine	fluconazole	erythromycin
nifedipine	itraconazole	troleandomycin
verapamil	ketoconazole	
	voriconazole	

Gastrointestinal Prokinetic Agents	Other Drugs	
cisapride	bromocriptine	nefazodone
metoclopramide	chloramphenicol	lansoprazole
	cimetidine	omeprazole
	cyclosporine	protease inhibitors
	danazol	ethinyl estradiol
	methylprednisolone	
	magnesium-aluminum-hydroxide	
	fluoroquinolones	

TABLE 3-4. Drugs That May Decrease Tacrolimus Blood Concentration

Anticonvulsants	Antimicrobials
carbamazepine	rifabutin
phenobarbital	caspofungin
phenytoin	rifampin

Herbal Preparations	Other Drugs
St. John's Wort	sirolimus

TABLE 3-5. Agents That Affect Cyclosporine Blood Concentration

Agent	CYP3A effect	P-glycoprotein effect	Cyclosporine blood concentration
Amiodarone		inhibits	increases
Clarithomycin	inhibits		increases
Diltiazem	inhibits	inhibits	increases
Erythromycin	inhibits	increases express	increases
	increases content		
Fluconazole	inhibits		increases
Grapefruit juice	inhibits		increases
Itraconazole	inhibits	inhibits	increases
Ketoconazole	inhibits	inhibits	increases
Nicardipine	inhibits	inhibits	increases
Verapamil	inhibits	inhibits	increases
Fluoroquinolones	inhibits	decreases express	increases
Carbamazepine	induces	induces	decreases
Phenobarbital	induces	induces	decreases
Phenytoin	induces	induces	decreases
Rifampicin	induces	inhibits	decreases

TABLE 3-6. Drugs That Affect Sirolimus Concentrations

Agent	Sirolimus blood concentration
Cyclosporine	increases
Diltiazem	increases
Ketoconazole	increases
Rifampicin	decreases

TABLE 3-7. Drugs That Affect Everolimus Concentrations

Agent	Everolimus blood concentration
Rifampicin	decreases
Rifabutin	decreases
Erythromycin	increases
Azithromycin	increases
Clarithromycin	increases
Telithromycin	increases
Itraconazole	increases
Voriconazole	increases
Fluconazole	increases
Ketaconazole	increases
Ritonavir	increases
High fat meal	decreases

Note: These tables are summaries of possible interactions. They do not include all possibilities.

OTHER FACTORS THAT CAUSE VARIATION IN DRUG BLOOD CONCENTRATION

Immunosuppressive drugs such as cyclosporine, tacrolimus, sirolimus, everolimus and MPA are lipophilic drugs. The extent of absorption through the intestinal membrane depends on several physicochemical properties including dissolution rate, particle size, polarity, and emulsion phase. Therefore, the type of oral formulation is critical. The same drug may display different absorption profiles depending on its formulation. This should be kept in mind, for instance, when switching from one formulation to another, including the use of different generic formulations.

Examples of some factors that could influence oral absorption include:

- Food: drug ingestion close to consumption of a meal may cause a delay in the time to peak concentration, a reduction of both the peak concentration and the AUC. The effect will be more pronounced for a high-fat meal than for a low-fat meal. This has been observed and well documented for calcineurin inhibitors, but not for MPA. The effect of food intake on oral drug absorption relative to the fasting state is shown in Figure 3-4.

- Time: it is recommended that immunosuppressive drugs be administered in a consistent manner, both with respect of the type of meal as well as timing of ingestion relative to consumption of the meal. Also, the AUC is higher in the morning (fasting state) than the evening.

- Diet: since 1991, it has been well known that grapefruit juice can inhibit both the efflux-transport-protein P-glycoprotein (P-gp) and the CYP3A4 enzymes in the enterocytes, resulting in an important increase of the drug blood concentration. The effect of grapefruit juice intake on oral drug absorption relative to the fasting state is also shown in Figure 3-4.

  St John's Wort (antidepressant herbal product) acts as an inducer of CYP3A and P-gp, causing a significant decrease of cyclosporine and tacrolimus AUC.

- Diarrhea: chronic diarrhea can reduce the P-gp activity in the GI tract and lead to an increase in the amount of tacrolimus reaching the blood circulation. This effect has not been reported for cyclosporine.

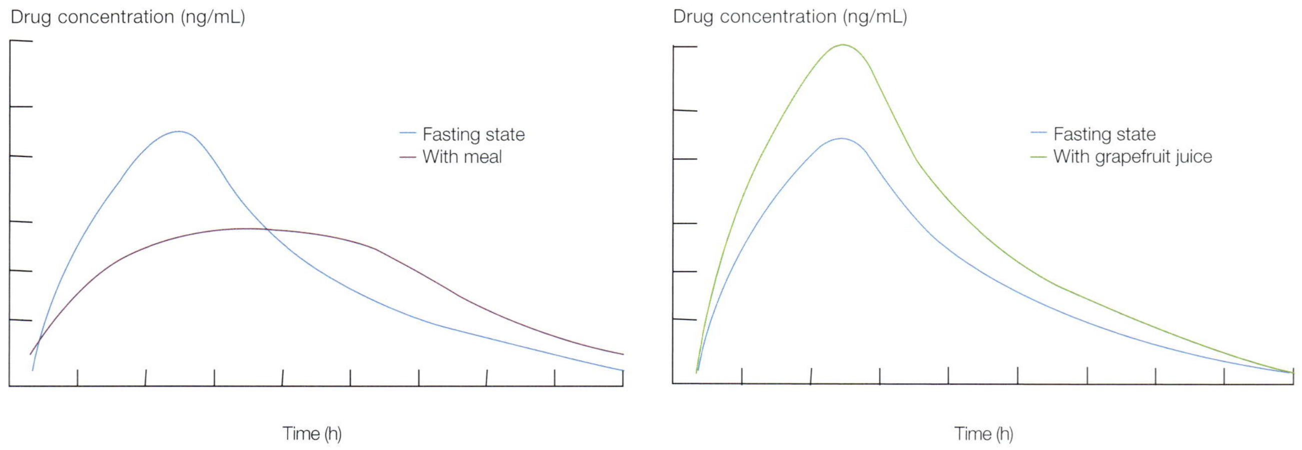

FIGURE 3-4. Different drug absorption profiles.

PHARMACOGENETICS

The science of pharmacogenetics links differences in gene structure (polymorphisms) with pharmacologic differences in drug metabolism, transport, or pharmacodynamic action. It is well recognized that different patients respond in a variety of ways to the same dose of the same medication. Immunosuppressive drugs are substrates of the enzymes (CYP3A4/5 for calcineurin inhibitors and mTOR inhibitors), and transporter proteins (P-gp, Multi-drug Resistance Protein 2 (MRP2)). These enzymes and proteins are subject to functional changes due to genetic polymorphisms, which can affect drug metabolism (Figure 3-5).

Single nucleotide polymorphisms (SNPs, Figure 3-6) in genes encoding biotransformation enzymes (*CYP3A*) and drug transporters (*ABCB1*) have opened up a promising way for the selection of individualized dosing. The relationship of these SNPs with immunosuppressive drug pharmacokinetics has been studied extensively after kidney, liver, heart, and lung transplantation. Part of the highly variable pharmacokinetics described above could, indeed, be explained by genetic polymorphisms of *CYP3A5* and *ABCB1*.

About 15-25% of Caucasians and 70% of African-Americans express CYP3A5 activity (*CYP3A5*1/*1 or *1/*3*) resulting in a two-fold higher drug clearance of tacrolimus. As a consequence, kidney transplant recipients expressing the enzyme require a 2-3 fold higher tacrolimus dose than non-expressers. Some authors propose a loading dose based on the pre-transplantation genetic polymorphism assessment, allowing patients to achieve target blood concentrations faster.

Liver transplantation poses its own problems, since it is necessary to take into account enzymes and protein activities both from the donor (liver) and the recipient (intestine).

Intracellular accumulation of drugs (e.g. in the lymphocytes), is associated with the pharmacodynamic activity of these drugs, and is also related to the expression of transporter proteins across the cell wall. On the other hand, patient susceptibility to long-term nephrotoxicity has been associated with some SNPs. Knowledge of these genetic traits could allow effective assessment of individual risk and selection of treatment according to patient parameters. Further studies are needed to provide evidence that a genetic analysis, combined with TDM, has the potential to optimize drug use and dosing after transplantation.

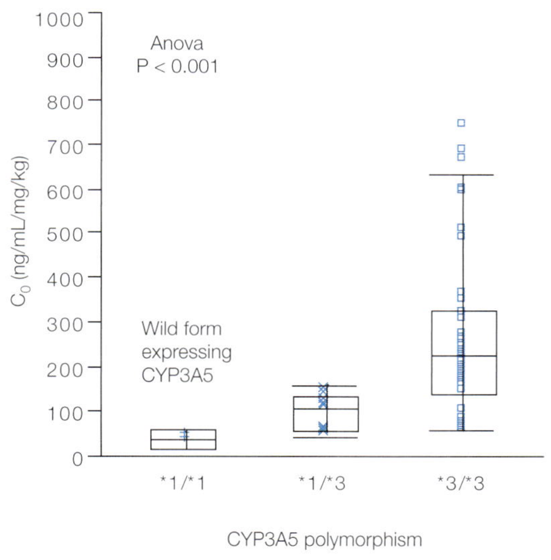

FIGURE 3-5. Effect of CYP3A5 polymorphism on dose and body weight adjusted tacrolimus through blood concentrations in a population of 50 kidney transplant patients. Data - Laboratory of Analytical Chemistry, Universitaires St. Luc, Brussels - unpublished.

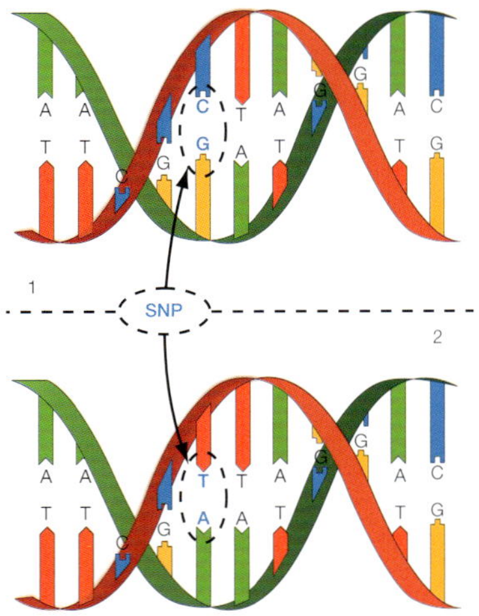

FIGURE 3-6. Most of the mutations observed involve Single Nucleotide Polymorphisms (SNPs).

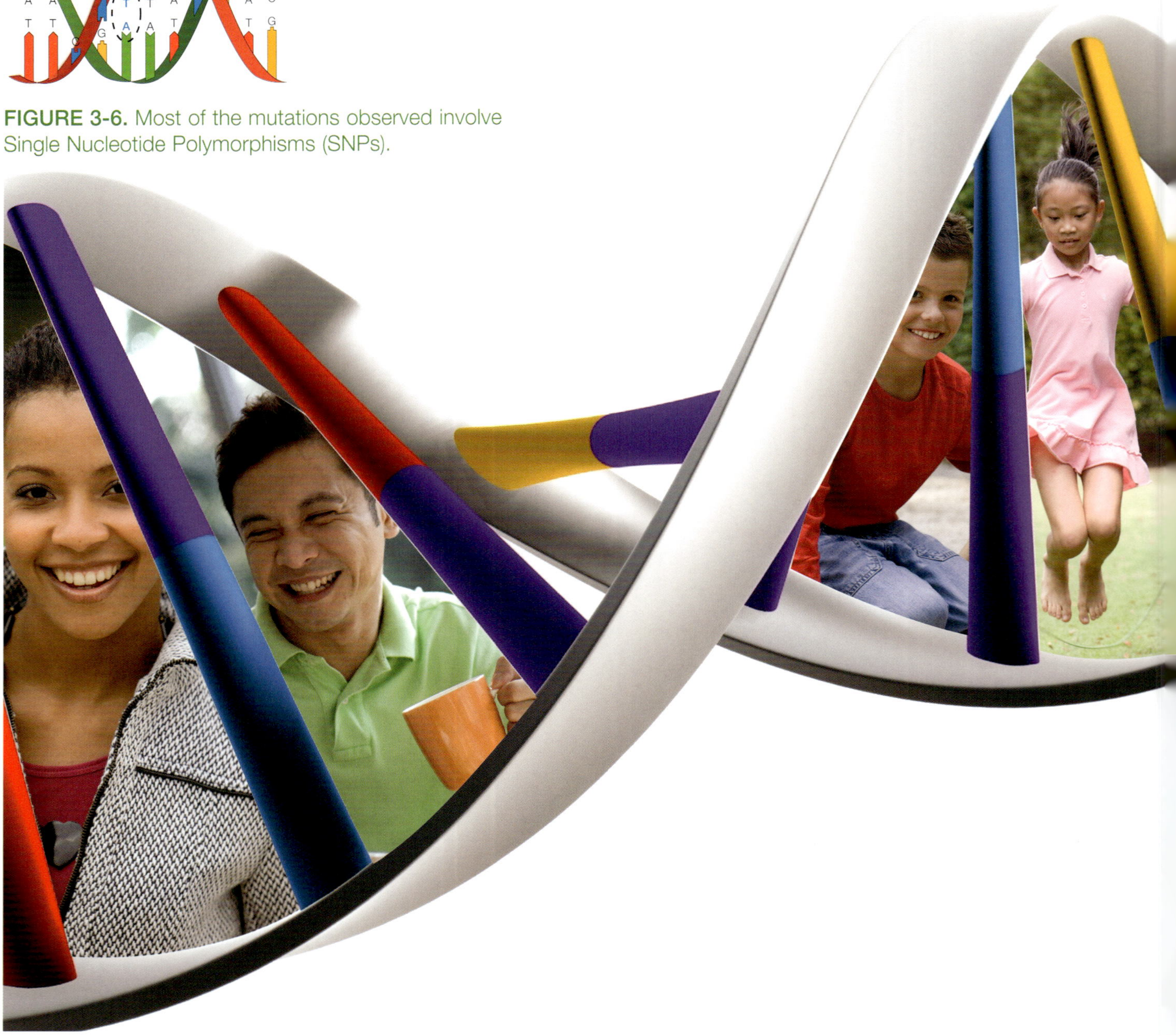

FIGURE 3-7. Visible ethnic phenotypic diversity parallels invisible ethnic metabolic genetic diversity.

THERAPEUTIC RANGES

Most transplantation centers use the whole blood trough concentration (C_0) to adjust drug doses, even though some controversies remain about the significant relationship between C_0 and clinical outcome. The full AUC is generally considered as the best marker of drug exposure, but it is rather difficult to obtain for a number of reasons. Unfortunately, C_0 does not always predict AUC accurately. Other strategies have been proposed to better estimate AUC:

- C_2 monitoring (sampling 2h after drug intake, well established for cyclosporine).
- Limited sampling strategies (involving generally 3 blood samples and a mathematical equation).
- Population pharmacokinetics together with Bayesian estimates.

Figure 3-8 below summarizes the commonly used sampling strategies for TDM.

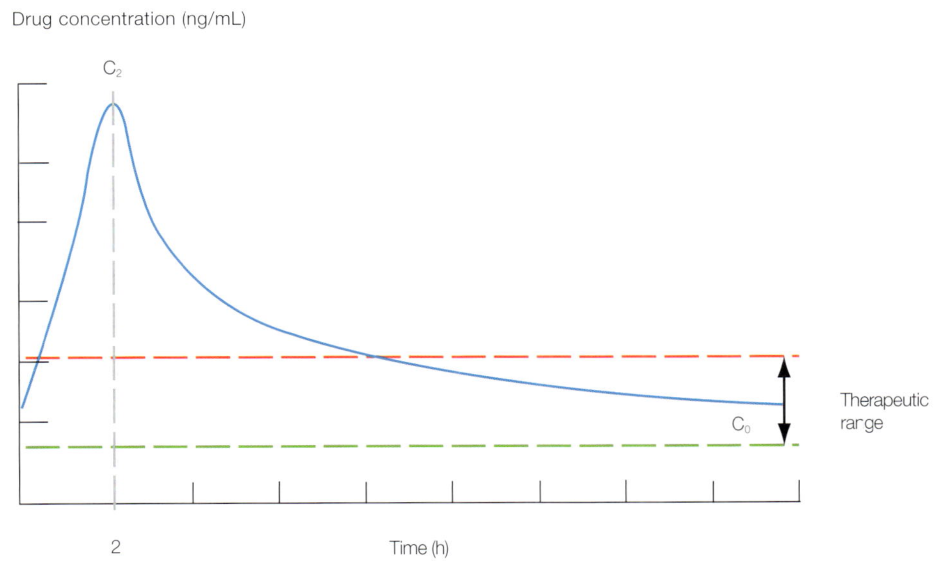

FIGURE 3-8. C_2, C_0 and AUC (Area Under Curve) as a function of time. C_2 may or may not be identical to C_{max}.

03 THERAPEUTIC DRUG MONITORING OF IMMUNOSUPPRESSIVE DRUGS

Providing recommendations for therapeutic ranges of immunosuppressive drugs is particularly difficult. Indeed, therapeutic ranges may depend on a large number of factors, including:

- Concomitant immunosuppressive protocols.
- Time post-transplantation.
- Type of organ transplanted.
- Age of the patient.
- Susceptibility to infection or adverse effects.

Moreover, it is important to emphasize the fact that drug concentrations in blood remain an indirect way to evaluate drug exposure, and that patient management should include other clinical or biological evaluations.

The current trend is to promote, as much as clinically feasible, dose minimization. Tacrolimus is a good example of this trend. In the early 1990s initial target ranges were kept above 15 ng/mL. As noted previously in Chapter 2 in the ELITE-Symphony study the best patient outcomes were observed with an immunosuppressive treatment involving low tacrolimus exposure (target blood concentrations 3-7 ng/mL), with MMF, steroids and IL2-mAb induction therapy. Tacrolimus minimization was associated with the lowest acute rejection rate (11.2%) and the best allograft function (65 mL/min, estimated mean GFR calculated from serum creatinine concentration) after 1 year.

The relationship found between blood concentrations of these immunosuppressants and clinical outcome (rejection and adverse effects) may vary from one study to another. This could be explained by:

- Different analytical methods.
- Different concomitant therapies.
- Different patient populations.
- Different recording techniques for, or definitions of, clinical outcomes.
- Different susceptibility of the patients to infection or adverse effects.

As a consequence, the therapeutic windows presented in Table 3-8 should be considered as concentration ranges displaying a low probability of adverse events.

TABLE 3-8. Suggested Therapeutic Ranges

Trough level	Time	Kidney	Liver	Heart or lung
Cyclosporine C_0 (C_2) (ng/mL)	Initiation Maintenance	150-250 (>1200) 75-150 (800)	250-350 (>1000) 100-200 (600)	250-350 150-250
Tacrolimus (ng/mL)	Initiation Maintenance Minimization	10-15 5-10 3-7	10-20 5-10 -	15-20 5-10 -
MPA (µg/mL)	Initiation Maintenance	1.3-3.5 (Cyclo) or 1.7-4.0 (Tac) Target AUC 30-60 µg.h/mL		
Sirolimus (ng/mL)	Initiation Maintenance	5-15		
Everolimus (ng/mL)	Initiation Maintenance	5-15 3-8		- 3-8, 3-12

ANALYTICAL TECHNIQUES FOR TDM OF IMMUNOSUPPRESSIVE DRUGS

Requirements for a TDM service

- There must be a reliable method to measure the drug.
- There must be data on the pharmacokinetics of the drug.
- There must be data to show that drug concentrations are related to the clinical effects of the drug.
- There must be defined times for sample collection.
- There should be good liaison between the laboratory and requesting clinicians.
- Sufficient data should be collected to allow for interpretation of the result.
- There should be a clear strategy for interpretation of the results.
- Periodically, there should be an audit of results to ensure that the service is suitable for current clinical demands.
- The laboratory providing the service to measure the drug should belong to an external proficiency testing scheme.

These considerations show clearly that TDM is a team activity. The maximum gain can only be achieved when an appropriate method is being used to measure the drug, when the laboratory, pharmacy and clinical staff have an understanding of the principles of pharmacokinetics, and when there are data on which to make the interpretation of the results. This integrated approach to the use of the data has led to the coining of the term *Therapeutic Drug Management*, implying more than just the measurement of drug concentrations, but also their interpretation in the context of the individual patient.

THE SAMPLE

Most TDM data for immunosuppressive drugs are based on pre-dose (trough) samples. There are other sampling strategies in use, for example, limited AUC sampling, and it is essential that sample timing in relation to the time of the last dose is recorded, to ensure the correct interpretation of the result.

Specific sample matrices are used for these assays. Whole blood samples must be well-mixed prior to analysis to ensure that there is no gradient of concentrations within the tube due to accumulation of the drugs within red blood cells.

The drugs are fairly stable in blood or plasma, with the exception of sirolimus, which is unstable at temperatures above about 30° C. This can have implications for sample transport in countries with high ambient temperatures. When samples are transported long distances for clinical studies or for TDM it is good practice to control the temperature. Once samples have arrived in the laboratory they should be stored in a refrigerator, at about 4° C, if they are not to be analyzed within a day. Samples that will not be analyzed for a week or more should be stored deep-frozen at -20° C or lower. All the drugs described here are stable through several freeze-thaw cycles.

CRITERIA FOR SELECTING AN ANALYTICAL METHOD

There are several reasons for choosing a particular analytical technique to implement in a laboratory. They include:

- What apparatus is available?
- Is suitable technical expertise available?
- Is the chosen technique suitable for its clinical purpose?
  - Does it have adequate sensitivity?
  - Is it selective for the drug of interest?
  - Can the result be provided in the turn-around-time required by clinicians?
- What are the capital and running costs?

There have been a number of consensus papers written on TDM of immunosuppressive drugs. These can be helpful in selecting an appropriate analytical technique when a laboratory is starting a TDM service, or intends to change methodology. Key papers are included in the Bibliography at the end of this chapter. Even when a method has been chosen, it is important to keep abreast of developments in methodology, as the availability of new assay methods may prompt a change in methodology. There may also be changes in prescribing practice which favor the performance of one method compared with another.

ANALYTICAL TECHNIQUES FOR TDM OF IMMUNOSUPPRESSIVE DRUGS

To measure cyclosporine and tacrolimus most laboratories are using an immunoassay; a minority of centers use chromatographic techniques. For the measurement of sirolimus, everolimus and MPA, depending on the local availability of some assays, laboratories are fairly evenly divided between immunoassay techniques and chromatographic techniques. Recently, an enzyme inhibition assay for MPA has also been released.

The relative use of each assay technique for the full range of drugs can be seen on the pages of the International Proficiency Testing Schemes website (see **Useful Websites**, at the end of this chapter). These schemes are used predominantly by laboratories in Europe, The Middle East and Australasia, but there are also participants in North and South America.

IMMUNOASSAYS

These assays are based on the affinity of the drug of interest for an antibody raised to recognize a portion of the molecule. The immunoassay techniques result in binding between drug in the clinical sample and the antibody in the test system. Since the amount of antibody is fixed, the amount of antibody-bound drug is related to the original concentration of the drug in the sample. The amount of antibody-bound drug is detected by the use of a label. In their simplest form, immunoassays allow drug in the sample to compete for antibody binding sites with a fixed amount of labeled drug. The labels include such things as a radio-isotope, an enzyme, a fluorescent compound or a magnetic particle.

A stylized representation showing the principles of an immunoassay is illustrated in Figure 3-9. As shown, the signal from the assay is plotted for a series of calibrators of known concentration. In the assay illustrated, the higher the drug concentration in the calibrator, the lower the signal. The concentration of drug in a clinical sample can be calculated by comparison with the calibration curve as shown in Figure 3-10.

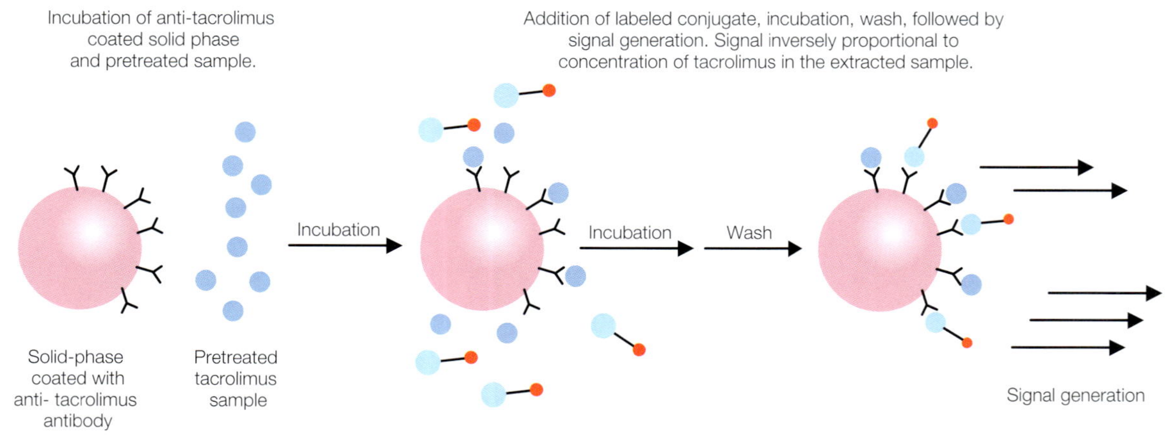

FIGURE 3-9. Principle of a competitive immunoassay for the measurement of tacrolimus concentration in whole blood.

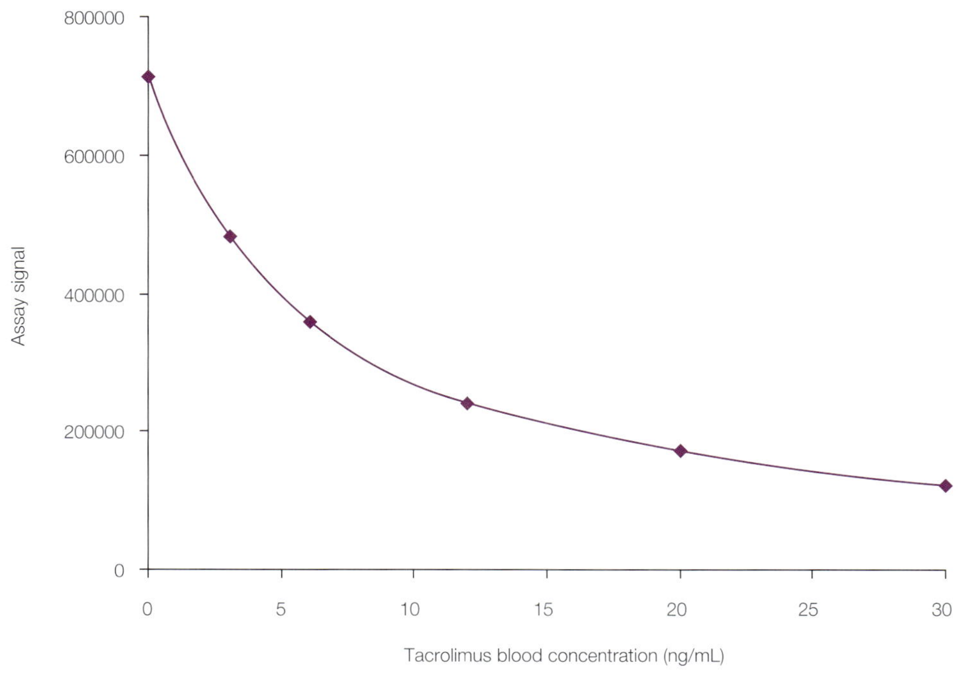

FIGURE 3-10. Tacrolimus calibration curve produced by an immunoassay technique.

Essentially, there are two main groups of immunoassay:

- Heterogeneous – the antibody-bound drug has to be separated from the unbound drug before the signal is measured.
- Homogeneous – the antibody-bound drug and the unbound drug do not need to be separated before the signal is measured.

Examples of the heterogeneous immunoassays include radioimmunoassays (RIA) and enzyme-linked immunosorbent assays (ELISA). Both techniques have been used to measure immunosuppressive drugs. Today they are little used to measure immunosuppressive drugs, in the case of RIA because of the growing unpopularity of using radio-labeled compounds.

The homogeneous assays are more easily automated, since the antibody-bound and unbound fractions do not need to be separated.

A number of assay technologies are in use for the immunosuppressive drugs. Examples of both homogeneous and heterogeneous assays include:

- Fluorescence Polarisation Immunoassay (FPIA).
- Microparticle Enzyme Immunoassay (MEIA).
- Chemiluminescent Microparticle Immunoassay (CMIA).
- Enzyme Multiplied Immunoassay Technique (EMIT).
- Affinity Column-Mediated Immunoassay (ACMIA).
- Cloned Enzyme Donor Immunoassay (CEDIA).
- Direct Chemiluminescence Immunoassay (CLIA).

These assays are performed on clinical analyzers which form part of the core apparatus of most clinical laboratories. As a result, the assays can usually be introduced without the need for large capital investment.

Immunoassays of this type are supplied with pre-prepared calibrators, so there is no necessity for the laboratory to purchase the drug and a suitable matrix in which to prepare the calibrators. In addition, diagnostics companies usually supply, or make available, a set of control samples which can be run as internal quality control samples in each assay.

Because cyclosporine, tacrolimus, sirolimus and everolimus are measured in whole blood, sample pre-treatment is needed to release the drug from the red cell. This step is usually performed before loading the samples onto the analyzer, but some assays are able to run the procedure as part of the automated assay.

As noted earlier, MPA is measured in plasma or serum. The target concentrations are much higher than those associated with the other four drugs (of the order 1-3 mg/L in pre-dose samples). Sample pre-treatment is not needed for any of the platform assays in current use, based on EMIT, CEDIA or enzyme immunoassay technology.

The main contentious issue with the use of immunoassays is the high probability that the antibody will cross-react with the metabolites of the drug of interest. As a result, immunoassays tend to give higher results than chromatographic techniques.

The bias introduced by cross-reactivity often results in the development of target concentration ranges that are specific to a particular assay. Users of immunoassays should be aware of any bias that can be introduced by cross-reactivity and of any clinical situations in which the bias could be increased. For instance, metabolite concentrations of cyclosporine and tacrolimus are much higher during periods of liver dysfunction. Assays that cross-react with these metabolites are likely to give higher results compared with those assays that cross-react less, or chromatographic assays. Typical results for cyclosporine are shown in Figure 3-11.

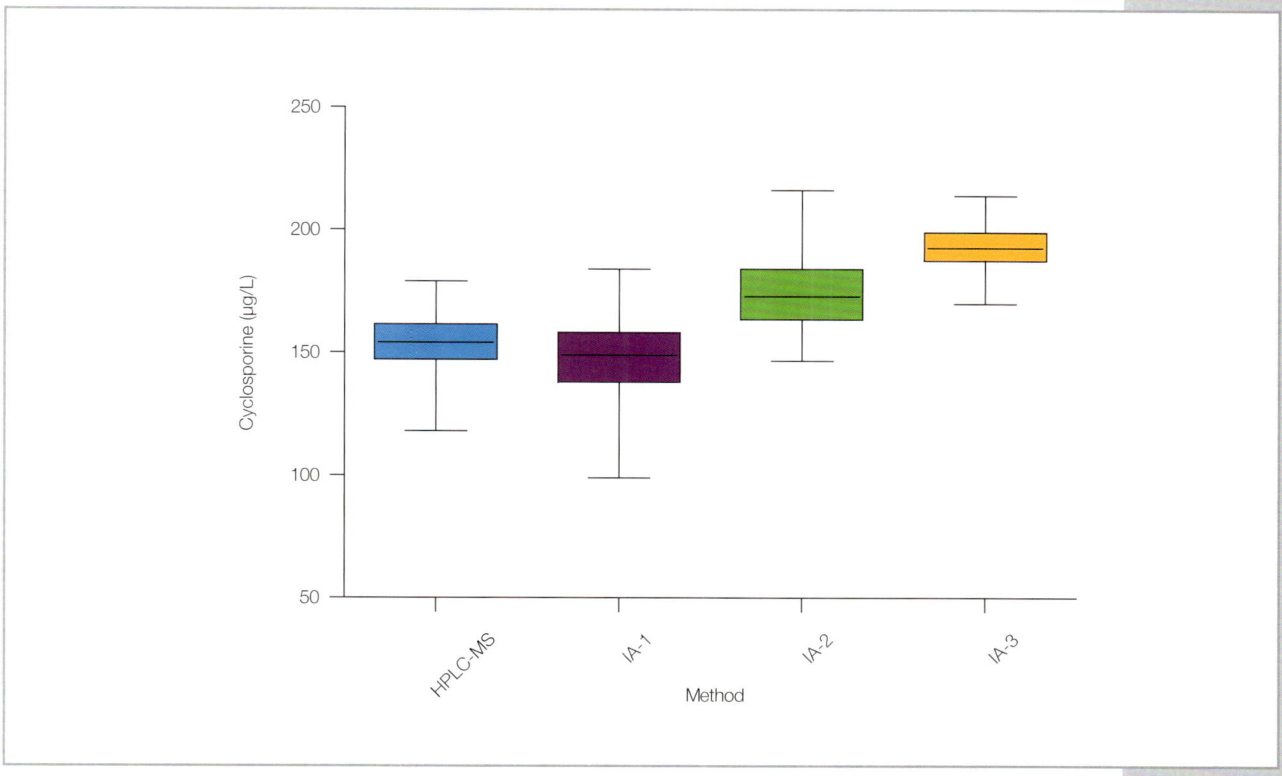

FIGURE 3-11. Results for the measurement of cyclosporine in a pooled blood sample from patients who had received the drug following liver transplantation.

HPLC-MS = high-performance liquid chromatography with mass-spectrometric detection, IA = immunoassay. The data are shown as box and whisker plots. The box is the inter-quartile range and the horizontal line in the box is the median. The whiskers show the upper and lower ranges. Two of the immunoassays show a positive bias relative to the chromatographic assay. The mean value for IA-3 was 26% higher than the mean value for the chromatographic assay. Data – International Proficiency Testing Scheme – unpublished.

It is particularly important that clinicians, who may move from one transplant center to another, are advised which method has been used to measure a drug, and whether the target range is influenced by the method used.

CHROMATOGRAPHIC ASSAYS

High-performance liquid chromatography (HPLC) is the chromatographic technique used to measure the immunosuppressive drugs. The fundamentals of the technique are illustrated in Figure 3-12.

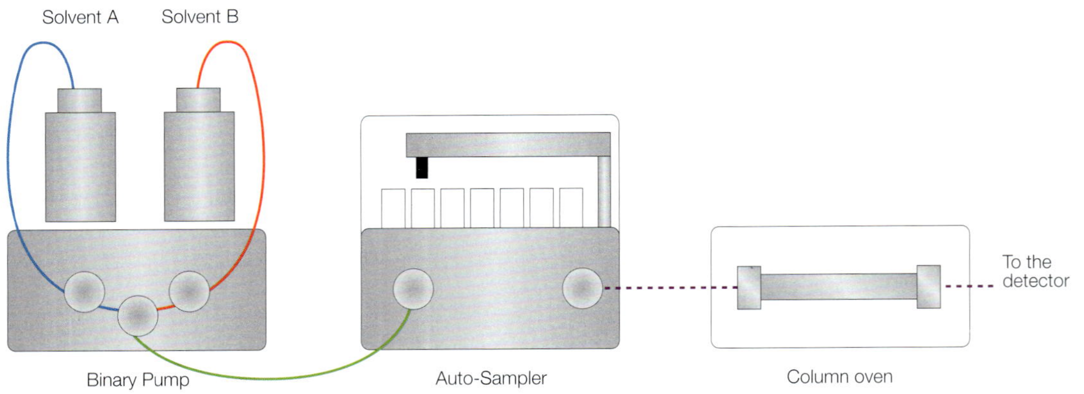

FIGURE 3-12. Schematic representation of an HPLC system.

The drug is first extracted into a suitable solvent and the extract injected onto the chromatographic column. Partition or absorption processes between the components of the sample extract and the particles of the analytical column (the stationary phase) then effect the separation of the substances in the extract, as they are eluted from the analytical column by the mobile phase. The separation of the components in the extract can be altered by the choice of solvents in the mobile phase. The eluate that emerges from the column must be monitored by a detection system and the quantity of the drug can be measured by integrating the area of the peaks detected, and comparing the area with those generated by a set of calibrators.

An internal standard, a compound structurally related to the drug being measured, is added to the sample to allow for any losses during the extraction procedure. The concentration of the drug is usually measured by measuring the peak areas for the drug and internal standard and comparing their ratio with the ratios produced for known calibrators, as shown in Figure 3-13.

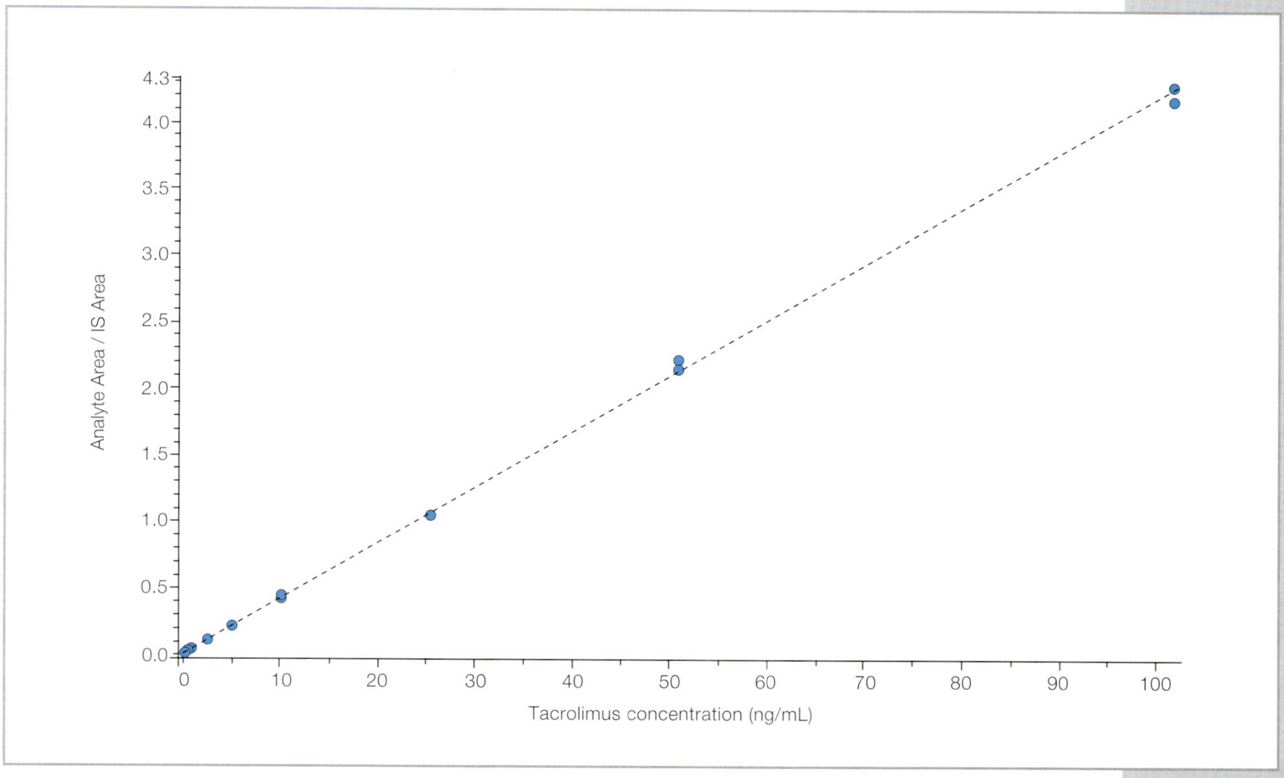

FIGURE 3-13. Calibration curve for the measurement of tacrolimus by HPLC-MS. The ratio for the peak area of tacrolimus and the peak area of the internal standard (IS), ascomycin, is plotted against the concentration of tacrolimus. Data-Analytical Unit, St. George's - University of London, on file.

When the various elements of the system – drug extraction, stationary phase of the analytical column, mobile phase and flow rate through the column – have been optimized, then the drug of interest should be resolved from the components of the matrix, metabolites of the drug and any other drugs likely to be given during routine therapy.

When cyclosporine was introduced some centers established HPLC assays with ultraviolet detection (HPLC-UV). The wavelengths employed for detection of the drug posed some challenges for the selectivity of the technique, since the drug has a large number of metabolites with the potential to elute close to the parent compound.

It is not possible to use UV detection to measure tacrolimus. Blood concentrations are much lower than for cyclosporine and the structure of the molecule makes UV detection impractical. Thus, all centers with HPLC assays for tacrolimus use mass-spectrometric detection.

This technique passes the column eluate into a mass analyzer, which is either tuned to look for the molecular ion of the drug of interest or a specific fragment of that molecular ion, formed in a second collision chamber (LC/MS or LC/MS/MS, respectively). A full-scan spectrum for sirolimus, showing the molecular ion and two of its daughter ions is shown in Figure 3-14.

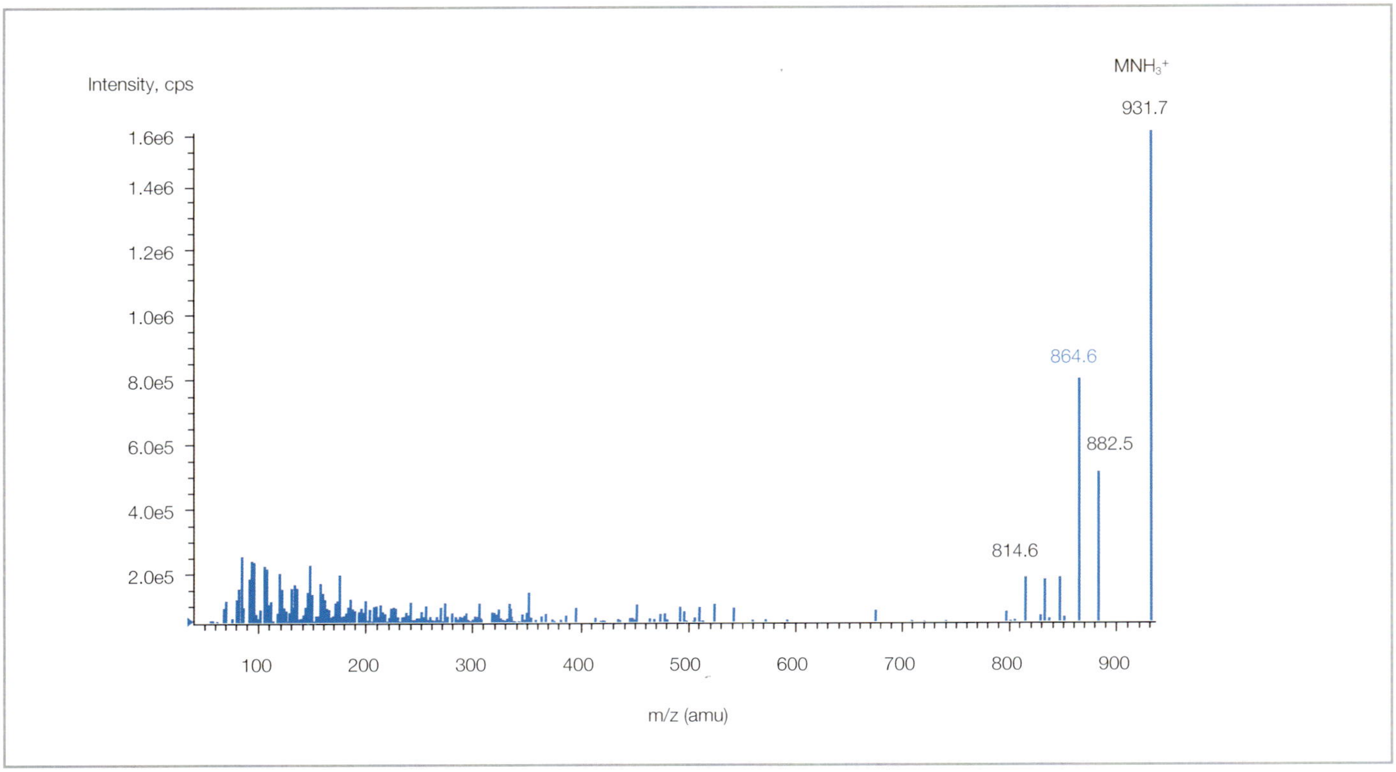

FIGURE 3-14. Full-spectrum ion scan for the measurement of sirolimus by mass-spectrometry. The figure shows the molecular ion of the ammonium adduct and the daughter ions. In practice, the ion used to quantify the drug is 864.6 m/z. m/z – mass to charge ratio. amu – atomic mass units. Data – Analytical Unit, St. George's – University of London, on file.

The technique has been particularly useful for the measurement of tacrolimus, sirolimus and everolimus, because of the low blood concentrations (of the order 2 – 20 ng/mL) associated with routine therapy. Assays have been described for both sirolimus and everolimus based on UV detection, but the chromatographic run times are relatively long and they are not as sensitive as the mass-spectrometric assays. The inherent advantages of mass-spectrometric assays are shown in Figures 3-15 and 3-16.

These show chromatograms for extracts of samples from a patient receiving sirolimus, using UV and MS/MS detection, respectively. It is clear that the mass-spectrometric assay is less prone to interference from other substances in the extract and that the compounds of interest, the drug and the internal standard, can be allowed to elute much faster from the column and still be free from interference.

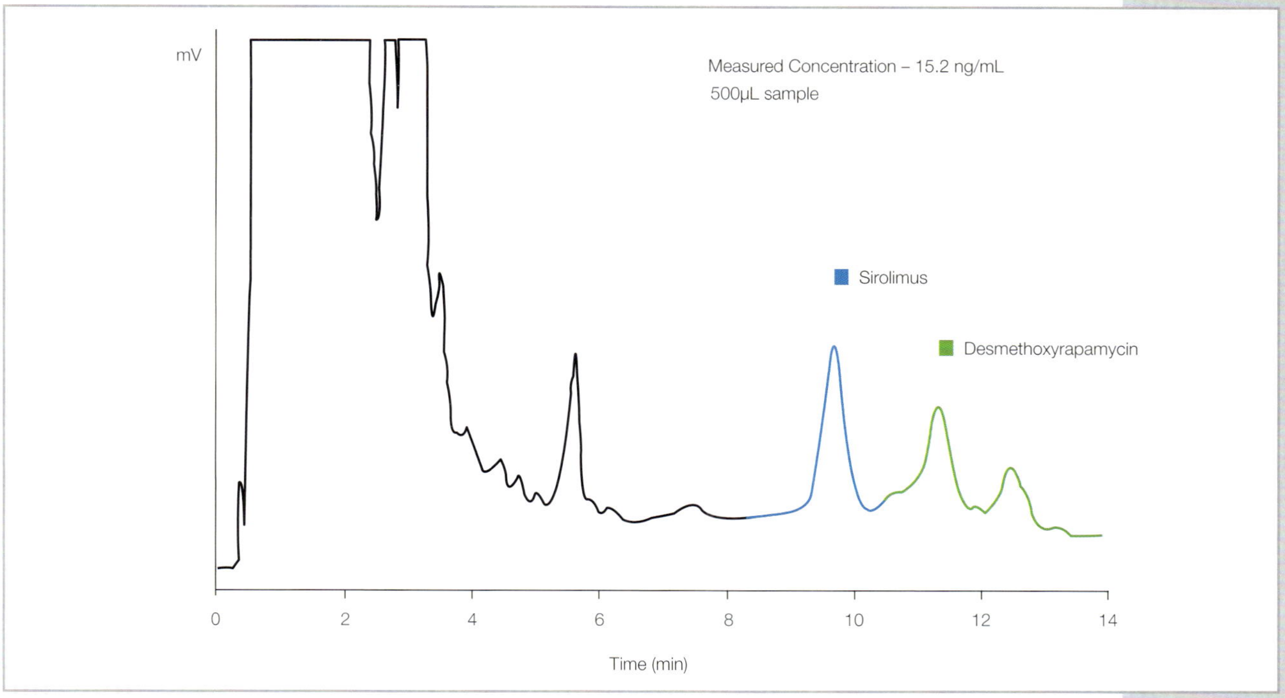

FIGURE 3-15. Chromatogram of extracted whole blood sample from a patient receiving sirolimus therapy following renal transplantation using HPLC with UV detection. Data-Analytical Unit, St. George's – University of London, on file.

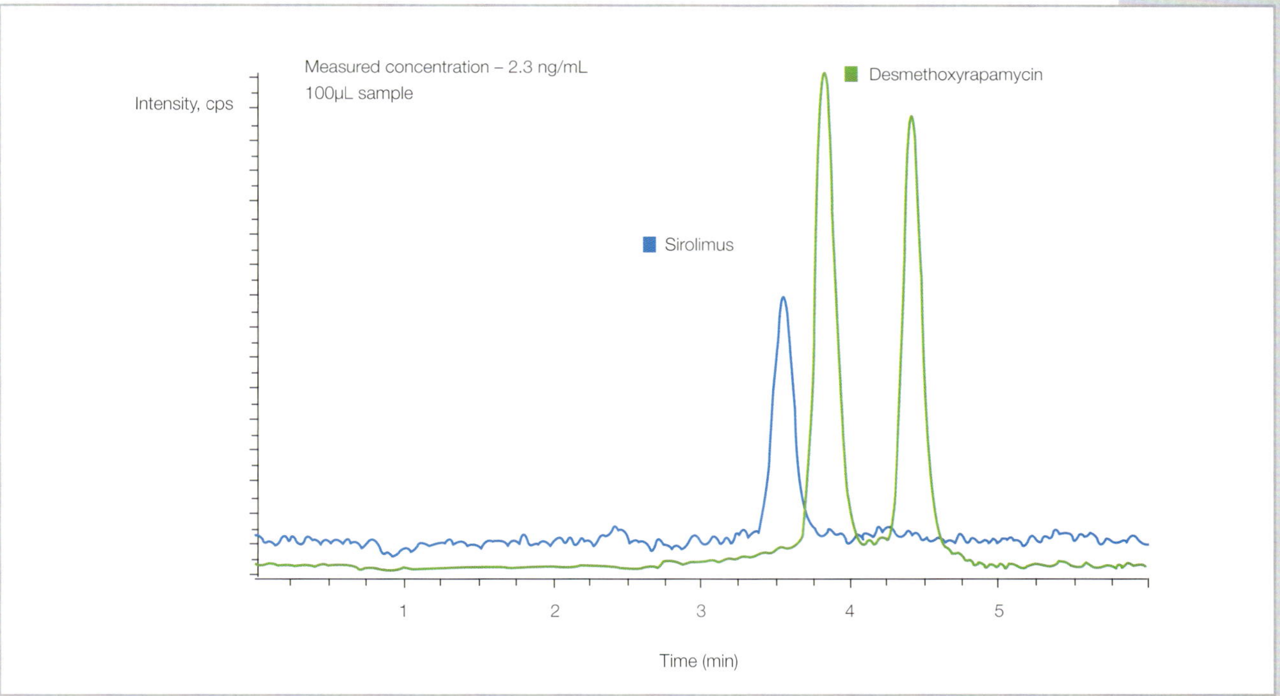

FIGURE 3-16. Chromatogram of extracted whole blood sample from a patient receiving sirolimus therapy following renal transplantation using HPLC with tandem mass-spectrophotometric detection. Data-Analytical Unit, St. George's – University of London, on file.

In addition, the sensitivity of mass-spectrometric assays is better, allowing the use of a smaller sample volume. Using this technique it is also possible to analyze a blood sample for several of the immunosuppressive drugs using a single injection of an extract, as shown in Figure 3-17.

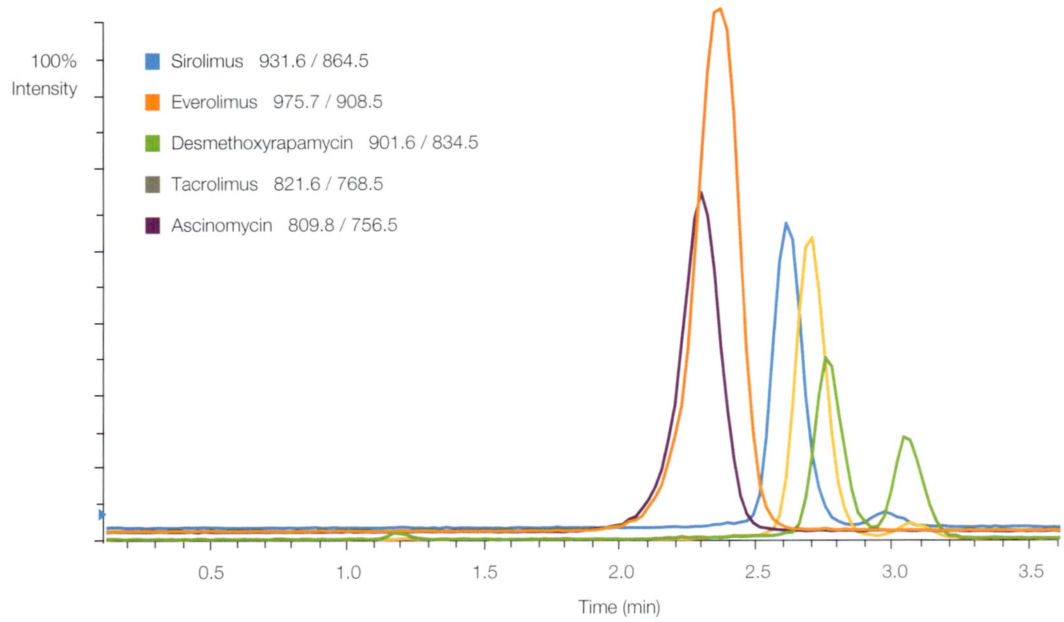

FIGURE 3-17. Chromatograms showing the ability of LC-MS to measure several drugs in one extract and one chromatographic run. Data – Analytical Unit, St. George's – University of London, on file. Desmethoxyrapamycin and ascomycin are used as internal standards. The numbers are the molecular ions and the product ions used for the measurements.

The enhanced sensitivity achieved by mass-spectrometric assays has opened up some research areas that would be difficult or impossible to pursue using immunoassays. For instance, assays have been described that are capable of measuring cyclosporine and tacrolimus in blood mononuclear cells. These assays are being used to compare whole blood concentrations with concentrations measured in the target cells.

Laboratories using chromatographic assays must obtain suitable calibrators for their assays. If prepared in-house, then a reference material with a certificate of analysis must be purchased. The resulting calibrators must be tested against previous batches, to ensure consistency, and against either an external control or controls prepared from a separate weighing of the reference material. The matrix in which the calibrators are prepared must also be representative of clinical samples and must be shown to be free of the target drug(s).

Chromatographic assays, even with mass-spectrometric detection, are not without their own problems. Similar to the immunoassays, there is the potential for interference from metabolites of the target drug. This has to be overcome by adequate chromatographic separation or by detection of fragments from the molecule that are selective for the parent compound. It is rarely possible to obtain pure standards of the metabolites to elute on the chromatographic system.

The choice of a suitable internal standard can also be difficult. Compounds structurally similar to the drug of interest may not be readily available. For mass-spectrometric detection a stable isotope labeled form of the target drug is the ideal choice. However, at the time of writing, the availability of internal standards labeled with atoms such as deuterium is limited. Two appropriate internal standards, for cyclosporine and everolimus, are available under the auspices of the International Association of Therapeutic Drug Monitoring and Clinical Toxicology – see **Useful Websites** at the end of this chapter.

The use of a stable isotope labeled internal standard helps to overcome one of the main problems of the mass-spectrometric assay – matrix effects. These are usually the consequence of short chromatographic run times, which allow substances in the matrix to suppress ionization of the target drug, resulting in erroneous results. If several drugs are analyzed in one chromatographic run it is important that appropriate internal standards are used for each drug.

IMMUNOASSAY OR CHROMATOGRAPHIC ASSAY?

Immunoassays are:

- easy to implement.
- suitable for batch analysis.
- have pre-prepared calibrators.

But they:

- are often subject to cross-reactivity with metabolites of the drug.
- may lack sufficient sensitivity for some drugs or applications.

Chromatographic assays are:

- potentially highly selective for the drug of interest.
- potentially highly sensitive.
- capable of measuring several drugs in a single sample extract and chromatographic run.
- likely to have a wider calibration range.

But they:

- require a higher level of technical input.
- require the preparation or purchase of calibrators.
- may be subject to substantial effects related to the sample matrix.

ASSAY VALIDATION

Chromatographic assays must be validated. There are standard, internationally accepted criteria, for this process published by the US Food and Drug Administration (FDA). The criteria can be downloaded from the FDA website – see **Useful Websites**.

The process of assay validation should establish:

- the assay is linear across the dynamic range to be used.
- the upper and lower limits of quantitation.
- precision data for within-assay and between-assay performance.
- the selectivity of the assay for the drug(s) of interest.
- the results produced by the new assay compared with other chromatographic and/or immunoassay techniques.

COMPARISON OF METHODS

Because of developments in assay techniques and changes in prescribing practices it may be necessary to evaluate a new method or compare two methods. There are well documented procedures to follow.

To compare two methods for the measurement of a drug concentration in clinical samples, guidelines are available from the Clinical Laboratory Standards Institute – see **Useful Websites**. These guidelines show the recommended number of samples that should be analyzed, the range of concentrations they should encompass and the number of replicate analyzes to perform.

The assays should be tested by using clinical samples that are representative of the patient population to be served. If, typically, the patient population includes those with major organ dysfunction, those with serious infections or pediatric patients, then samples from these groups should be included, rather than just those from clinically stable patients.

There are a number of ways to analyze the data on comparative assay performance. The simplest is a linear regression analysis, but the analysis can be disproportionately influenced by high concentration values. A number of statistical tools are available to take into account factors such as variability in both the reference and test methods, and non-normal distribution of the data. These methods include Deming regression, Passing-Bablok regression and the Bland-Altman plot. An example of data analyzed by both simple linear regression and by a Bland-Altman plot is shown in Figures 3-18 and 3-19, respectively.

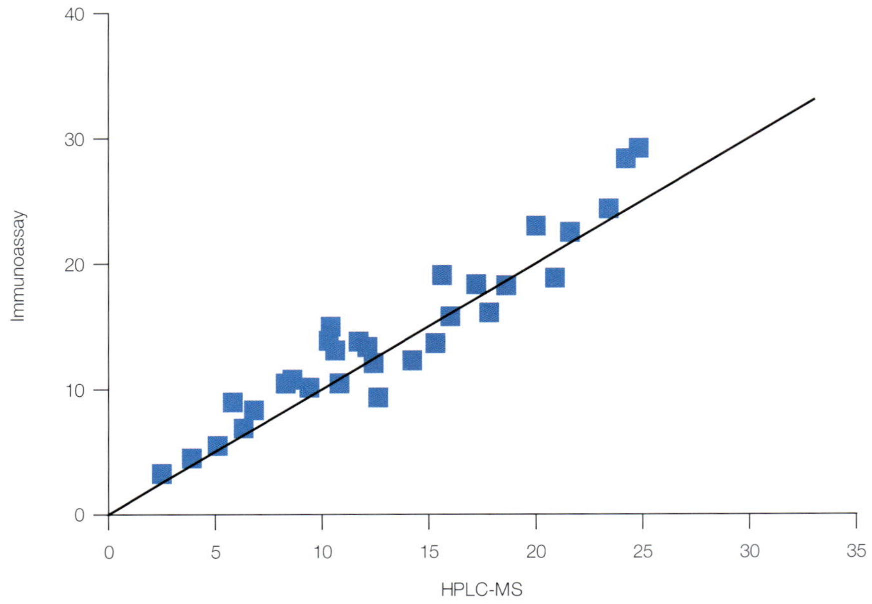

FIGURE 3-18. Method Comparison: Immunoassay versus HPLC-MS Linear Regression Plot. Linear regression analysis for the measurement of sirolimus in blood samples from 30 patients who had received the drug following kidney transplantation. The concentration (ng/mL) of sirolimus was measured by both HPLC-MS and an immunoassay. The line is the line of identity. There is a good correlation between the methods, correlation coefficient r = 0.95, but the data are significantly different from the line of identity. Data – Analytical Unit, St George's – University of London, on file.

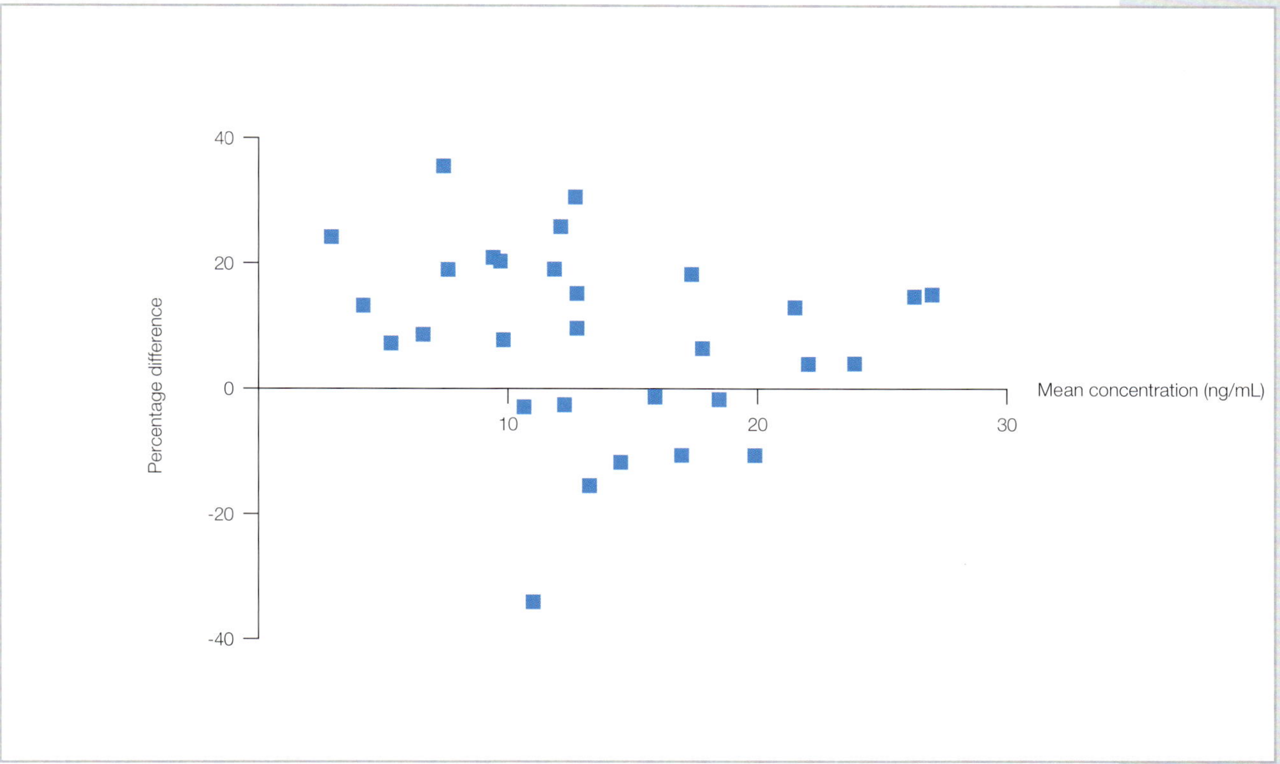

FIGURE 3-19. Method Comparison: Immunoassay versus HPLC-MS Bland-Altman Plot. The same data as shown in Figure 3-18 displayed as a Bland-Altman difference plot. Good agreement between methods would appear as a tight cluster of points around the horizontal line. There is a clear difference between the assays, especially at the lower concentrations.

If you purchase an assay kit the manufacturer will provide performance data with the package documentation and you should look to see if the device has been approved by a local regulatory authority, such as the FDA.

However, it is the responsibility of the user to ensure that the kit is performing within the specified limits and that the particular clinical application for which it is used does not compromise the performance. For instance, the sample matrix should be the one recommended for the assay.

Assay parameters that should be checked in-house are:

- Reproducibility, measured by coefficient of variation, at concentrations representative of clinical decision points.
- Sensitivity, by repeated measurements of a sample containing a low concentration and one that is drug-free for the drug of interest.
- Day-to-day performance should be recorded for the quality control samples and the results plotted using an appropriate software package.
- Long-term performance by participation in an external proficiency testing scheme.

Chromatographic assays developed in house require more extensive testing as noted above under **Assay Validation**. Even when a chromatographic assay has been validated, data on day-to-day performance should be collected and the assay should be challenged periodically to test the sensitivity and specificity of the technique.

PROFICIENCY TESTING

Laboratories providing TDM services for the immunosuppressive drugs should belong to a proficiency testing scheme. The schemes provide blinded samples which test a number of assay parameters and enable laboratories to compare their results with those obtained by other centers measuring these drugs.

In addition to some schemes run within individual countries there are two large international schemes. Details of their activities can be accessed on-line using the addresses shown under **Useful Websites**.

Proficiency testing schemes allow participants to compare the precision and accuracy of their method with other methods for the same drug. It is important to test both of these parameters.

Precision describes how closely a series of measurements of the same material are in agreement. It is important for the long-term use of the assay, facilitating confidence in the use of on assay. Precision is usually expressed as the percentage standard deviation of the mean (percent coefficient of variation). The precision of an assay is likely to vary across the dynamic range of the assay.

Accuracy describes the deviation of the result from the true value. However, there is, at present, no accepted reference standard for the true value for any of the immunosuppressive drugs. The parameter is usually described by the percentage deviation from the mean value produced by an accepted chromatographic assay. Accuracy is important when data are pooled, for instance when results from multiple sites are compared. If the methods do not produce the same numeric value, decision lines on treatment could be different between the various centers. The relationship between accuracy and precision is shown in Figure 3-20.

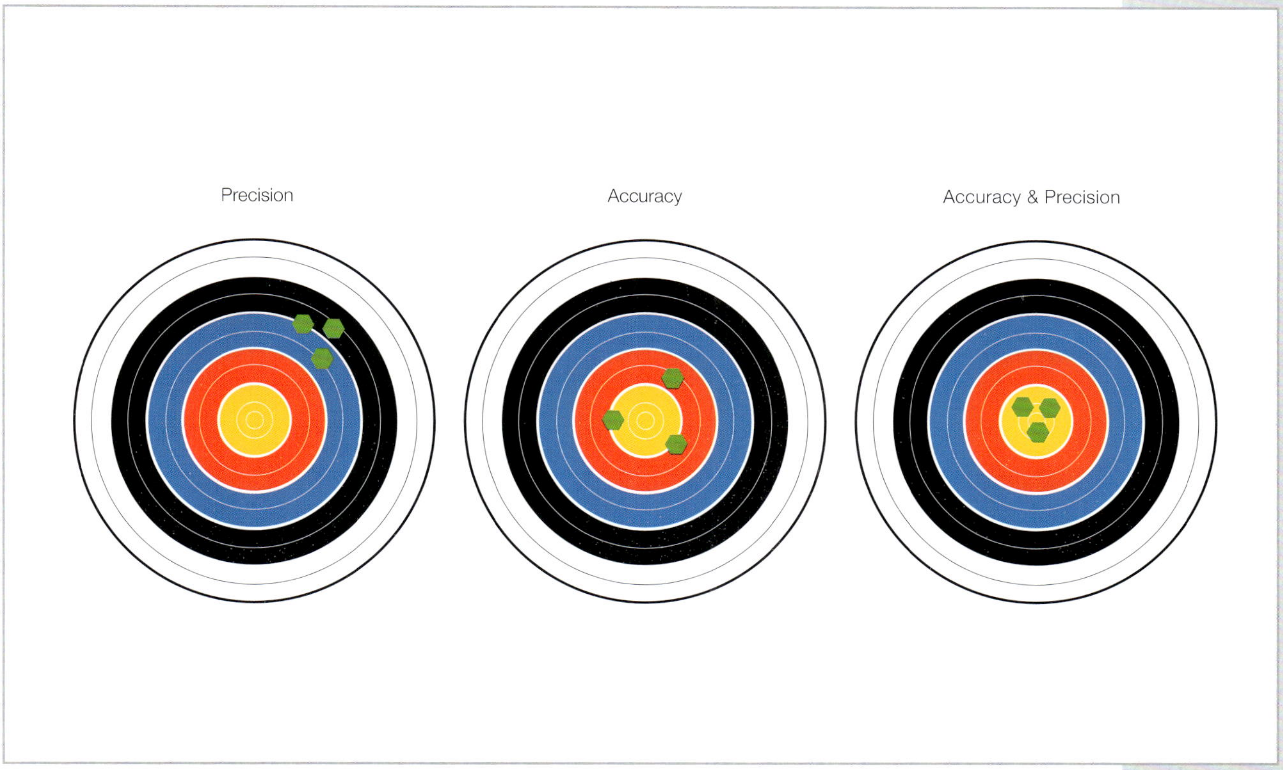

FIGURE 3-20. Relationship between accuracy and precision.

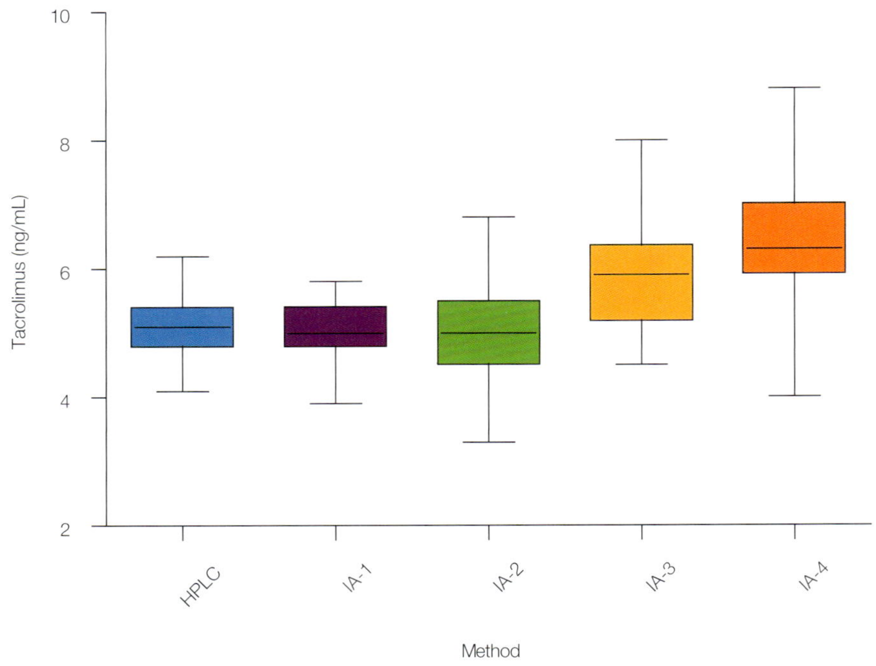

FIGURE 3-21. Results for the measurement of tacrolimus in a tacrolimus-free blood sample spiked with the drug to a final concentration of 5 ng/mL. Abbreviations and description of the plots same as for Figure 3-11. Two of the immunoassays have a positive bias compared with the chromatographic assay; IA-4 has a mean bias of 32% compared with the chromatographic assay. Data – International Proficiency Testing Scheme – unpublished.

The two concepts of precision and accuracy are illustrated in Figure 3-21 showing data for the measurement of tacrolimus. It is clear that for this sample, with a weighed in value of 5 ng/mL, three assays show good agreement with this value (good accuracy) but the dispersion of results is very wide for three of them (poor precision).

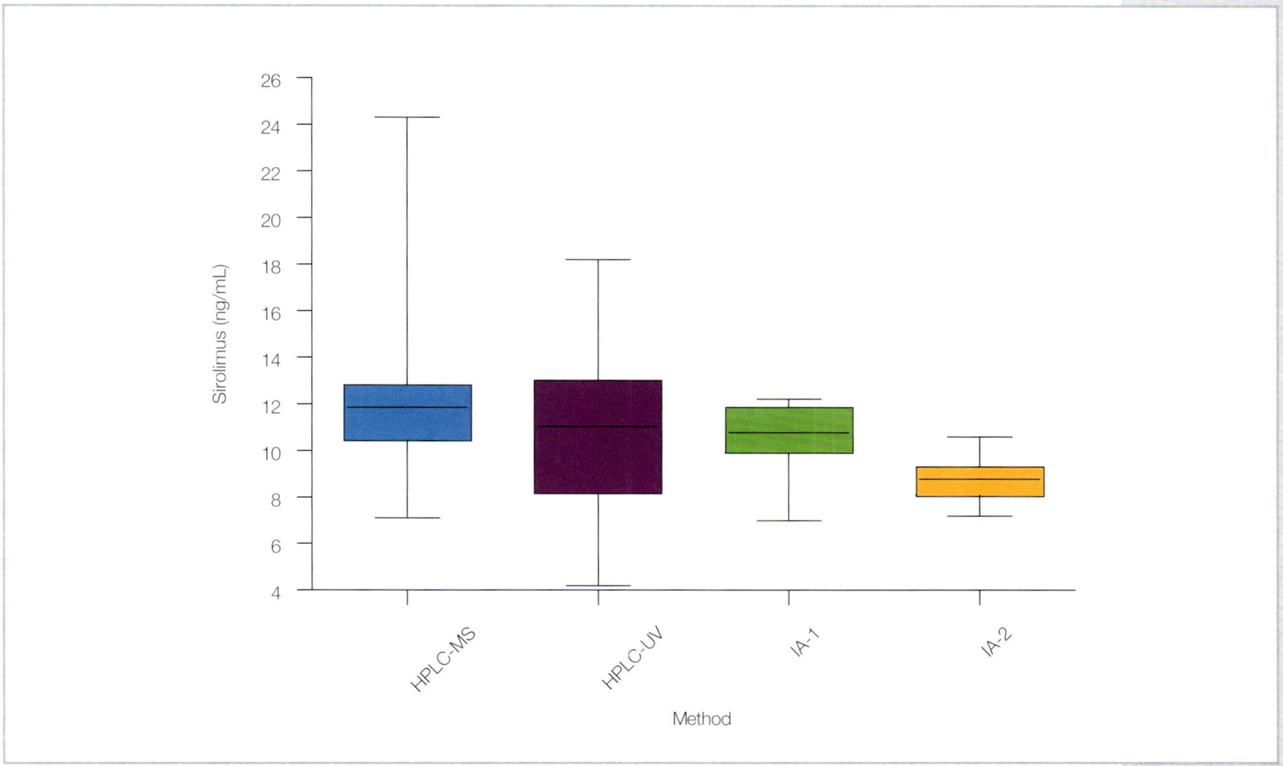

FIGURE 3-22. Results for the measurement of sirolimus in a sirolimus-free blood sample spiked with the drug to a final concentration of 11 ng/mL. Abbreviations and description of the plots as for Figure 3-11. IA-2 has a mean negative bias of 25% compared with the HPLC-MS assay. The HPLC-UV assay shows poor precision. Data – International Proficiency Testing Scheme – unpublished.

The impact that accuracy can have on the relative performance of an assay is illustrated in Figures 3-22 and 3-23. In Figure 3-22, results for the measurement of sirolimus show good agreement with the weighed-in value of 11 ng/mL for the two chromatographic assays and immunoassay 1, but immunoassay 2 shows a mean value about 20% below the target value. When these same assays are used to measure sirolimus in a pooled sample from patients receiving the drug (see Figure 3-23) the assays are in reasonable agreement. However, both immunoassays are affected by cross-reactivity; in the case of immunoassay 2 this has been masked by its low calibration bias.

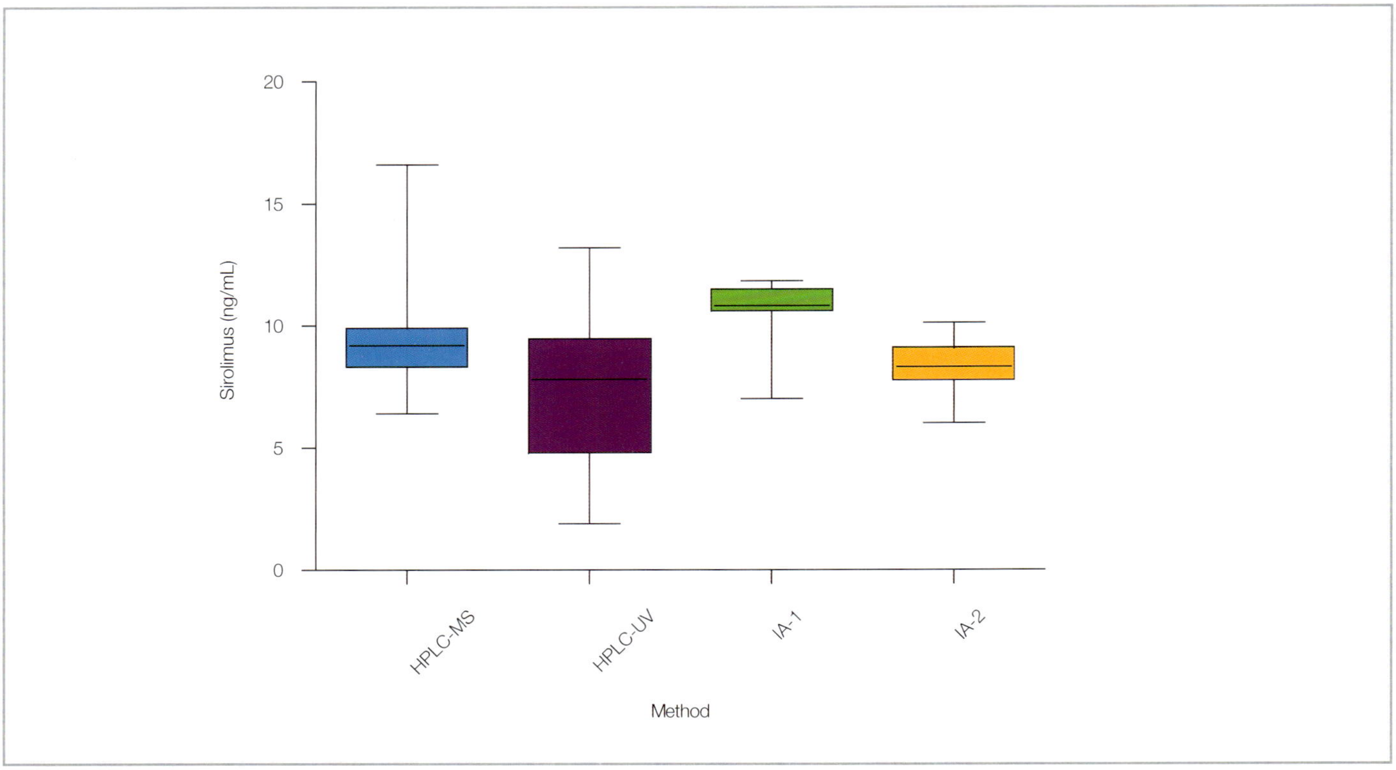

FIGURE 3-23. Results for the measurement of sirolimus in a pooled blood sample from patients who had received the drug following kidney transplantation. The same assays were used as those shown in Figure 3-22. Both immunoassays show a positive bias compared with the chromatographic assays, most likely due to cross-reactivity with metabolites of the drug. The bias with IA-2 is masked by its calibration bias. Data – International Proficiency Testing Scheme – unpublished.

Of course, proficiency testing is only a "snap shot" of assay performance. It only tests part of the total testing process, which also encompasses pre-analytical and post-analytical factors. It is no substitute for day-to-day quality control and laboratories must consider whether the frequency of proficiency testing is adequate for assays that are offered on a daily basis.

FACTORS TO CONSIDER WHEN INTERPRETING RESULTS

Measuring the drug is only part of the TDM process. All immunosuppressive drug measurements must be interpreted and not just viewed as a number, in isolation. The drug concentration is just one part of the decision tree for dose adjustment. The interpretation should take into account factors such as:

- The clinical indication for the use of the drug.
- The duration of therapy.
- Dose frequency.
- The time the sample was collected after the last dose.
- The method used to measure the drug.
- Other drug therapy.
- Clinical chemistry data relating to such factors as organ function and infection.
- Symptoms and signs of drug efficacy or toxicity.

The unthinking use of "therapeutic ranges" or "target concentrations" should be discouraged.

CONCLUSIONS

To provide a TDM service for immunosuppressive drugs:

- Select a method appropriate for your clinical needs.
- Ensure day-to-day performance by the use of suitable quality control material.
- Test the comparative performance of the assay by participation in an external proficiency testing scheme.
- Develop a clear strategy for using the results in collaboration with your clinical staff.
- Act on the result.
- Institute an audit system to test the validity of the target ranges used.

USEFUL WEBSITES

Analytical Services International Ltd, providers of proficiency testing schemes for immunosuppressive drugs. http://www.bioanalytics.co.uk

College of American Pathologists, providers of proficiency testing schemes for immunosuppressive drugs. http://www.cap.org

International Association of Therapeutic Drug Monitoring and Clinical Toxicology (IATDMCT), an association devoted to issues relating to TDM, in particular immunosuppressive drugs. http://www.iatdmct.org

Therapeutic Drug Monitoring, an international journal publishing on all aspects of TDM. Free on-line access is available to members of IATDMCT. http://www.drug-monitoring.com

Clinical Chemistry, an international journal publishing on many aspects of drug measurement and laboratory management. http://www.clinchem.org

Clinical and Laboratory Standards Institute, an organization which provides laboratory manuals on testing assay performance. http://www.clsi.org

FDA guidelines on chromatographic assay validation, essential reading when establishing and validating an assay. http://www.fda.gov/CDER/GUIDANCE/4252fnl.pdf

BIBLIOGRAPHY FOR CHAPTER 3

General papers on TDM of immunosuppressive drugs

Wallemacq P, Armstrong VW, Brunet M, Haufroid V, Holt DW, Johnston A, Kuypers D, et al. Opportunities to optimize tacrolimus therapy in solid organ transplantation: report of the European Consensus Conference. Ther Drug Monit. 2009;31:139-52.

Holt DW, Denny K, Lee TD, Johnston A. Therapeutic monitoring of sirolimus: Its contribution to optimal prescription. Transplant Proc. 2003;35:157S-161S.

Holt DW, Armstrong VW, Griesmacher A, Morris RG, Napoli KL, Shaw LM. International Federation of clinical chemistry/international association of therapeutic drug monitoring and clinical toxicology working group on immunosuppressive drug monitoring. Ther Drug Monit. 2002;24:59-67.

Van Gelder T, Le Meur Y, Shaw LM, Oellerich M, DeNofrio D, Holt C et al. Therapeutic drug monitoring of mycophenolate mofetil in transplantation. Ther Drug Monit. 2006;28:145-54.

Cole E, Midtvedt K, Johnston A, Pattison J, O'Grady C. Recommendations for the implementation of Neoral C(2) monitoring in clinical practice. Transplantation 2002;73:S19-S22.

Useful papers on HPLC methodology

Taylor PJ. Internal standard selection for immunosuppressant drugs measured by high-performance liquid chromatography tandem mass spectrometry. Ther Drug Monit. 2007;29:131-2.

Taylor PJ. High-performance liquid chromatography-mass spectrometry in the clinical laboratory. Ther Drug Monit. 2005;27:689-93.

Taylor PJ. Matrix effects: the Achilles heel of quantitative high-performance liquid chromatography-electrospray-tandem mass spectrometry. Clin Biochem. 2005;38:328-34.

Sauvage FL, Gaulier JM, Lachâtre G, Marquet P. Pitfalls and prevention strategies for liquid chromatography-tandem mass spectrometry in the selected reaction-monitoring mode for drug analysis. Clin Chem. 2008;54:1519-27.

McKeown DA, Lee TD, Holt DW. Therapeutic Drug Monitoring: Measurement of Immunosuppressants Using HPLC with Mass Spectrometric Detection. The Encyclopedia of Mass Spectrometry. Amsterdam: Elservier; 2006;813-823.

Capron A, Lerut J, Verbaandert C, Mathys J, Ciccarelli O, Vanbinst R, Roggen F, De Reyck C, Lemaire J, Wallemacq PE. Validation of a liquid chromatography-mass spectrometric assay for tacrolimus in liver biopsies after hepatic transplantation: correlation with histopathologic staging of rejection. Ther Drug Monit. 2007;29:340-8.

A paper describing the latest platform assay for tacrolimus.

Wallemacq P, Goffinet JS, O'Morchoe S, Rosiere T, Maine GT, Labalette M, Aimo G, et al. Multi-site Analytical Evaluation of the Abbott ARCHITECT Tacrolimus Assay. Ther Drug Monit. 2009;31:198-204.

Recent clinical studies relevant to TDM

Le Meur Y, Büchler M, Thierry A, Caillard S, Villemain F, Lavaud S, Etienne I, Westeel PF, de Ligny BH, Rostaing L, Thervet E, Szelag JC, Rérolle JP, Rousseau A, Touchard G, Marquet P. Individualized mycophenolate mofetil dosing based on drug exposure significantly improves patient outcomes after renal transplantation. Am J Transplant. 2007;7:2496-503.

Van Gelder T, Silva HT, de Fijter JW, Budde K, Kuypers D, Tyden G, Lohmus A, Sommerer C, Hartmann A, Le Meur Y, Oellerich M, Holt DW, Tönshoff B, Keown P, Campbell S, Mamelok RD. Comparing mycophenolate mofetil regimens for de novo renal transplant recipients: the fixed-dose concentration-controlled trial. Transplantation. 2008;86:1043-51.

Fine RN, Becker Y, De Geest S, Eisen H, Ettenger R, Evans R, Rudow DL, McKay D, Neu A, Nevins T, Reyes J, Wray J, Dobbels F. Nonadherence consensus conference summary report. Am J Transplant. 2009;9:35-41.

General papers

Bekersky I, Dressler D, Mekki QA. Effect of low- and high-fat meals on tacrolimus absorption following 5 mg single oral doses to healthy human subjects J Clin Pharmacol. 2001;41:176-83.

Baraldo M, Furlanut M. Chronopharmacokinetics of cyclosporin and tacrolimus. Clin Pharmacokinet. 2006;45:775-88.

Bekersky I, Dressler D, Mekki Q. Effect of time of meal consumption on bioavailability of a single oral 5 mg tacrolimus dose. J Clin Pharmacol. 2001;41:289-97.

Hebert MF, Park JM, Chen YL, Akhtar S, Larson AM. Effects of St John's wort (hypericum perforatum) on tacrolimus pharmacokinetics in healthy volunteers. J Clin Pharmacol. 2004;44:89-94.

Maes BD, Lemahieu W, Kuypers D, Evenepoel P, Coosemans W, Pirenne J, Vanrenterghem YF. Differential effects of diarrhea on FK506 versus cyclosporine A trough levels and resultant prevention of allograft rejection in renal transplant recipients. Am J Transplant. 2002;2:989-92.

Lemahieu W, Maes B, Verbeke K, Rutgeerts P, Geboes K, Vanrenterghem Y. Cytochrome P450 3A4 and P-glycoprotein activity and assimilation of tacrolimus in transplant patients with persistent diarrhea. Am J Transplant. 2005;5:1383-91.

Staatz CE, Tett SE, Clinical pharmacokinetics and pharmacodynamics of mycophenolate in solid organ transplant recipients. Clin Pharmacokinet. 2007;46:13-58.

Staatz CE, Tett SE, Clinical Pharmacokinetics and pharmacodynamics of tacrolimus in solid organ transplantation. Clin Pharmacokinet. 2004;43:623-53.

Kirchner GI, Meier-Wiedenbach I, Manns MP. Clinical pharmacokinetics of everolimus. Clin Pharmacokinet. 2004;43:83-95.

MacDonald A, Scarola J, Burke JT, Zimmerman JJ. Clinical pharmacokinetics and therapeutic drug monitoring of sirolimus. Clin Therapeutics. 2000;22:B101-B121.

Kim JS, Aviles DH, Silverstein DM, Leblanc PL, Matti Vehaskari V Effects of age, ethnicity and glucocortocoid use on tacrolimus pharmacokinetics in pedatric renal transplant patients. Pediatr Transplantation. 2005;9:162-9.

Hesselink DA, van Gelder T, van Schaik RH. The pharmacogenetics of calcineurin inhibitors: one step closer toward individualized immunosuppression. Pharmacogenomics. 2005;6:323-37.

Haufroid V, Wallemacq P, VanKerckhove V, Elens L, De Meyer M, Eddour DC, Malaise J, Lison D, Mourad M. CYP3A5 and ABCB1 polymorphisms and tacrolimus pharmacokinetics in renal transplant candidates: guidelines from an experimental study. Am J Transplant. 2006;6:2706-13.

Mourad M, Wallemacq P, De Meyer M, Malaise J, De Pauw L, Eddour DC, Goffin E, Lerut J, Haufroid V. Biotransformation enzymes and drug transporters pharmacogenetics in relation to immunosuppressive drugs: impact on pharmacokinetics and clinical outcome. Transplantation. 2008;85:S19-24.

Holt DW, McKeown DA, Lee TD, Hicks D, Cal P, Johnston A. The relative proportions of sirolimus metabolites in blood using HPLC with Mass-spectrometric detection. Transplant Proc. 2004;36:3223-5.

Christians U, Pokaiyavanichkul T, Chan L. Tacrolimus. Applied Pharmacokinetics & Pharmacodynamics. Principles of Therapeutic Drug Monitoring. M Burton, L Shaw, J Schentag, W Evans. Fourth Edition. 2006. Lippincott Williams and Wilkins. 530-562.

Strom T, Haschke M, Zhang YL, Bendrick-Peart J, Boyd J, Roberts M, Arabshahi M, Marbach P, Christians U. Identification of everolimus metabolite patterns in trough blood samples of kidney transplant patients. Ther Drug Monit. 2007;29:592-9.

The management of transplant recipients requires a carefully coordinated approach between the patient, clinician, pharmacist, and laboratorian to maintain the quality of life of the allograft recipient. As we have seen in the previous chapters, medical professionals are working together to ensure long-term survival of both their patients and their allografts. The following cases are actual medical cases we have encountered over the years in our profession and illustrate the complexity of the issues we face in obtaining the right balance between adequate levels of immunosuppression and prevention of disease.

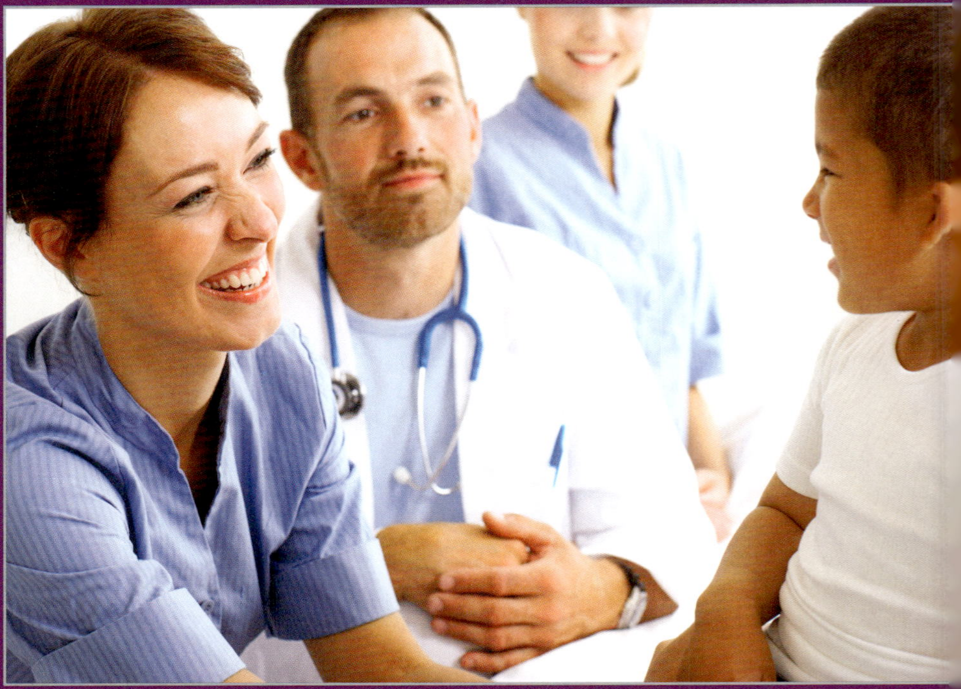

CHAPTER 4 CONTENTS

CASE HISTORY 1: CONVERSION FROM CYCLOSPORINE C_0 TO C_2 MONITORING AND THE EFFECT ON RENAL FUNCTION

Heart Transplant Recipient

- 42 year old female underwent heart transplantation in 1988 for viral cardiomyopathy.
- Treated with cyclosporine Neoral 200 mg bid (twice daily), Cellcept 1 g bid and Prednisone 5 mg od (once daily) as maintenance therapy.
- Heart function was excellent with no episodes of rejection.
- Cyclosporine dose was reduced to 150 mg bid to maintain a C_0 of 125 ng/mL.
- Serum creatinine at one year post-transplant was 1.1 mg/dL (97.2 µmol/L).

Two years later:

- At 2 years post-transplant the serum creatinine increased to 1.48 mg/dL (130.8 µmol/L).
- Cyclosporine dose was reduced to 100 mg bid.
- At 3 years post-transplant her creatinine had increased to 1.79 mg/dL (158.2 µmol/L).

Question: What is the appropriate management of this patient?

A) Continue to reduce cyclosporine
B) Switch to sirolimus
C) Switch to tacrolimus
D) Adopt C_2 monitoring

Answer: A) and D) Dose adjustment using C_2 monitoring

- A C_2 concentration was obtained and found to be 2100 ng/mL.
- Dose of CsA was reduced to 50 mg bid in a step-wise fashion to achieve a C_2 target of 800 ng/mL.
- At 6 months post-conversion from C_0 to C_2 monitoring:
  – no episodes of rejection.
  – serum creatinine fell to 1.5 mg/dL (132.6 µmol/L).
- At one year post-conversion to C_2 monitoring the serum creatinine was maintained at 1.18 mg/dL (104.3 µmol/L).

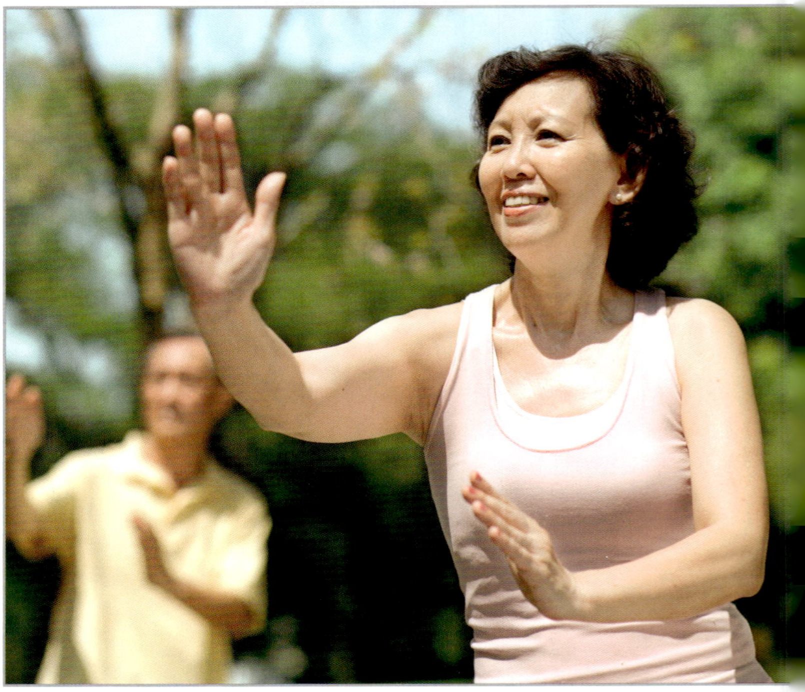

CASE HISTORY 2: CONVERSION FROM TACROLIMUS TO CYCLOSPORINE FOR PATIENT WITH HCV INFECTION: ADJUSTMENT OF DRUG CONCENTRATIONS AND EFFECT ON RESPONSE TO ANTI-VIRAL THERAPY

Patient with HCV Disease

- A 50-year-old male born in Poland in 1946 to Jewish Holocaust survivors.
- Immigrated into Canada in 1949.
- Father died of liver cirrhosis.
- Married with 2 daughters.
- PhD in Psychology.
- First seen in 1986 – diagnosed with non-A, non-B hepatitis based on laboratory abnormalities.
- No drug history, no alcohol ingestion.
- Risk factor – born in concentration camp and received vaccination.
- Returned for visit in 1989 with clinical deterioration; skin rash on legs, abnormal blood film with lymphocyte abnormalities.

Clinical and Laboratory Findings

Physical examination
- Hepatosplenomegaly.

Ultrasound
- Nodular, coarse liver with enlarged spleen, no ascites.

Infection status
- HBsAg negative, anti-HAV positive.

Laboratory findings

• AST	192 IU/L
• Bilirubin	1.8 mg/dL (30.8 μmol/L)
• ALP	198 IU/L
• INR	1.1
• Hb	121 g/L (12.1 g/dL)
• WBC	2.8 x 10^9/L
• Platelets	110,000 x 10^9/L

Question: Which test/s is appropriate?

A) Skin biopsy

B) 24 hour urine collection

C) Serum cryoglobulins

D) All of the above

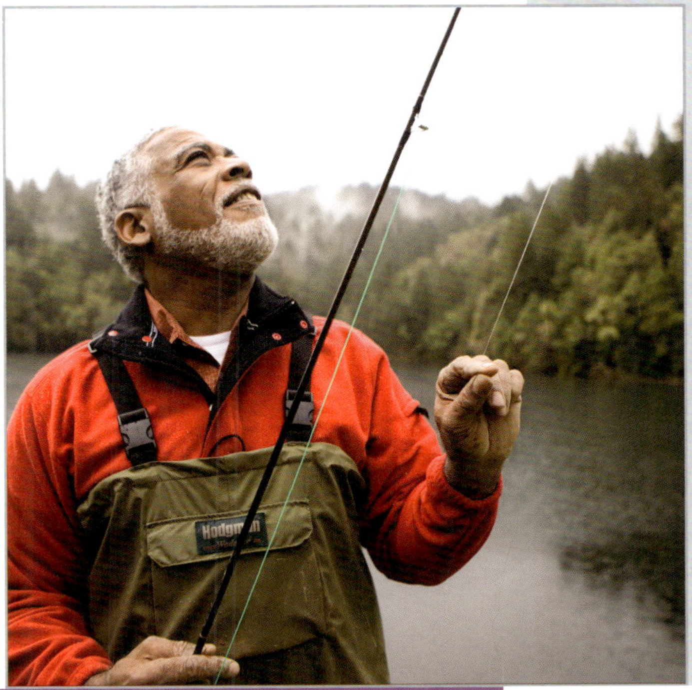

Answer: D) All of the above

Test results

- Cryoglobulins positive.
- Skin biopsy showed immune complex disease.
- Urine protein 2.8 g/L (0.28 g/dL).
- Urinalysis compatible with membranoproliferative glomerulonephritis.

Clinical course

- Returned to clinic with ascites.
- Bilirubin 5.0 mg/dL (86 µmol/L)
- INR 2.8
- WBC 2.6
- Platelet count 40,000 x 10^6/L
- AST 229 IU/mL
- ALT 304 IU/mL

Question: What is an appropriate next step?

A) Treatment with interferon and ribavirin

B) List for transplantation

C) Neither of the above

Answer: B) List for transplantation

Patient underwent orthotopic liver transplantation and was treated with an immunosuppressive regimen including tacrolimus. The explanted liver was showing cirrhosis as indicated in Figure 4-1.

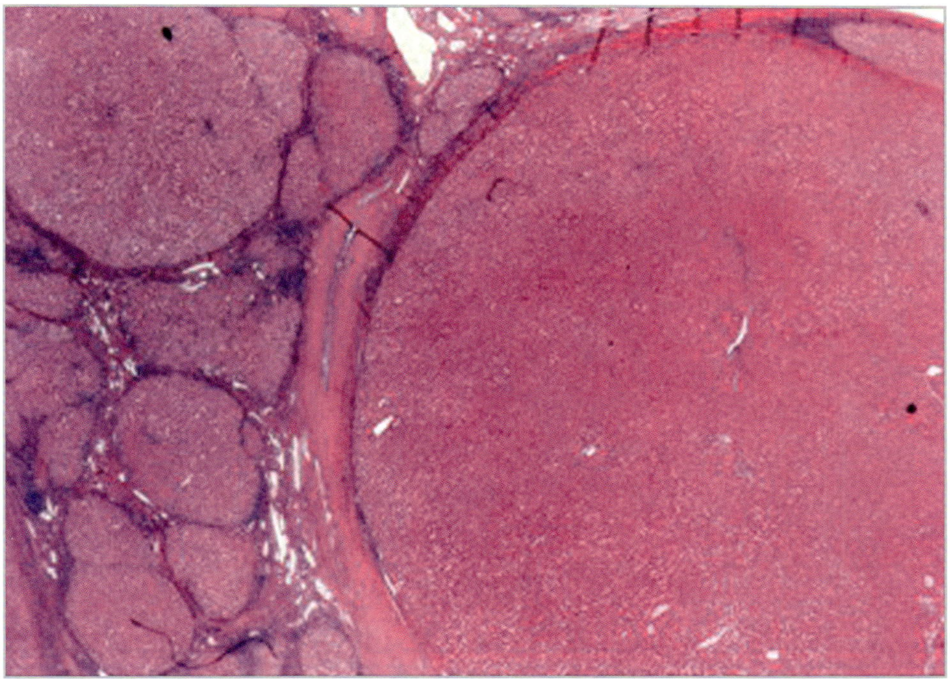

FIGURE 4-1. Explanted liver showing cirrhosis with regenerating nodules and dysplasia (magnification x400)

Patient was monitored post-transplant for serum Glutamic Oxalocetic Transaminase (AST), Total Bilirubin (T Bili), and creatinine (Cr) as shown in Figure 4-2. The serum concentration of both AST and T Bili increased from Day 28 to 2 months post-transplant.

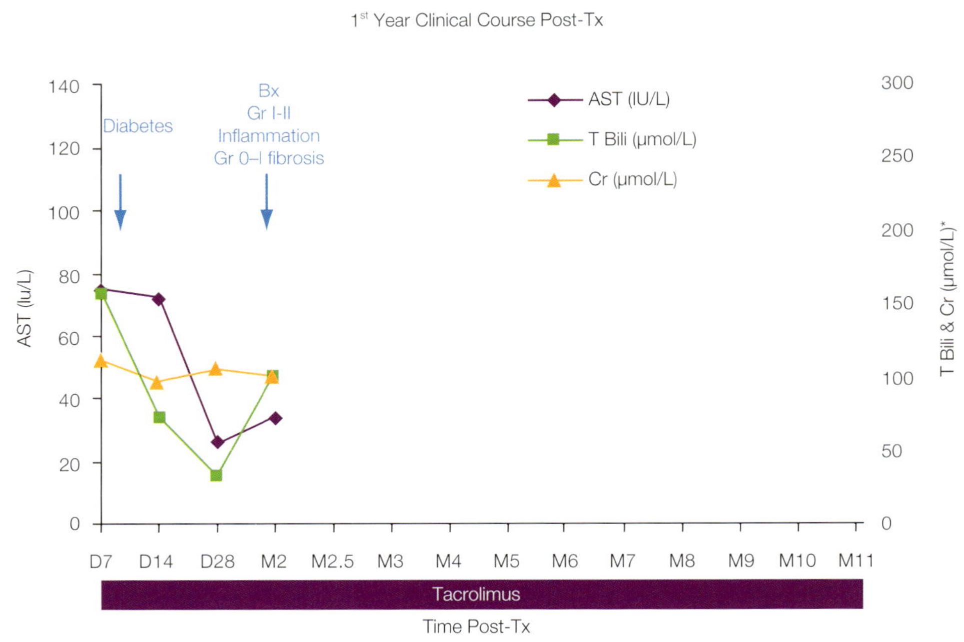

* Creatinine 1 mg/dL = 88.4 µmol/L; Bilirubin 1 mg/dL = 17.1 µmol/L

FIGURE 4-2. Clinical course of the liver transplant recipient during tacrolimus immunosuppressive therapy.

The increase in the serum concentration of AST and T Bili at month 2 was investigated and a liver biopsy was performed with the results shown in Figure 4-3.

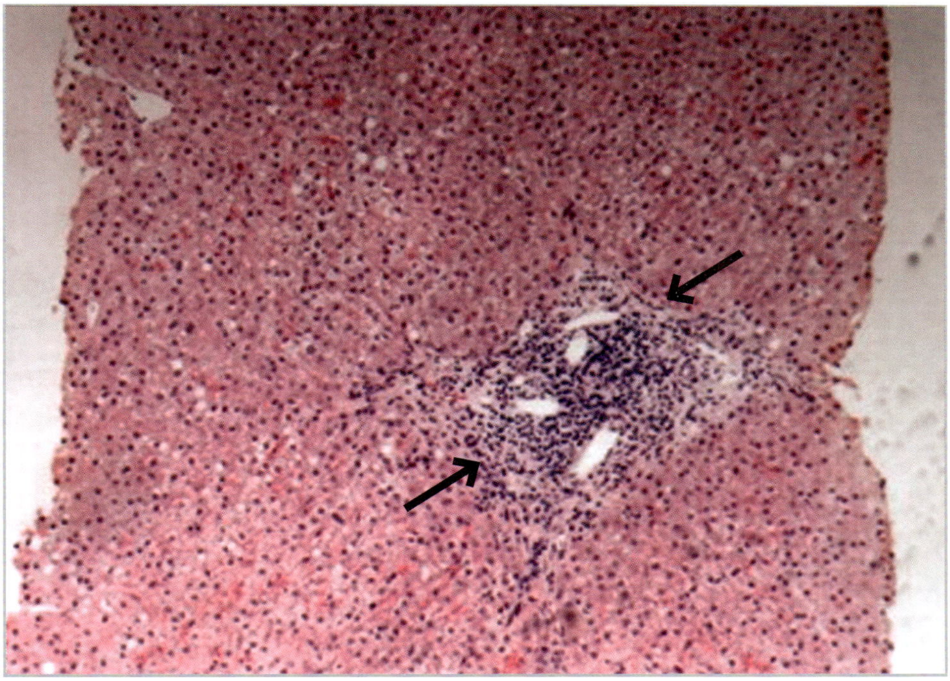

FIGURE 4-3. Liver biopsy (Hematoxylin (H) and Eosin (E)) showing evidence of mild recurrent HCV with portal infiltrate (arrow) (magnification x200).

Recurrent HCV infection was treated with interferon and ribavirin (Rebetron®) and another liver biopsy was performed to assess the status of the HCV infection as shown in Figure 4-4.

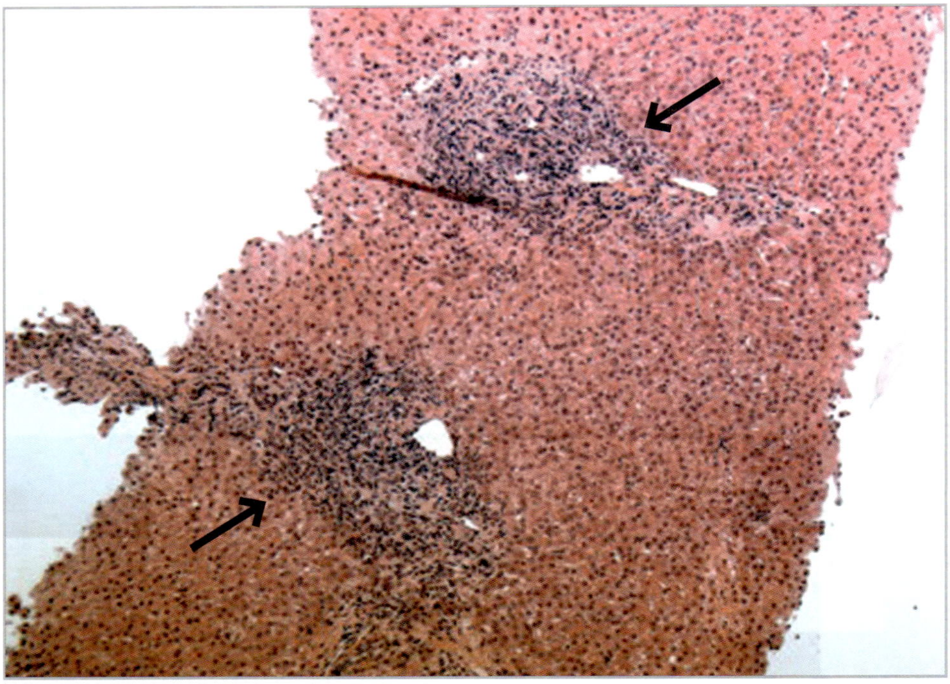

FIGURE 4-4. Post-Rebetron liver biopsy (H&E) showing moderate to severe recurrent HCV disease with portal infiltrate (arrow) and increased hepatic fibrosis (magnification x200).

Question: What is the appropriate next step?

A) Continue present regimen

B) Switch to cyclosporine

C) Switch to cyclosporine and consider retreatment with Rebetron

Answer: C) Switch to cyclosporine and consider retreatment with Rebetron

Patient was switched from tacrolimus to cyclosporine therapy and monitored for serum AST, T Bili, and creatinine as shown in Figure 4-5. The serum concentration of AST decreased from Day 12 to Day 15 following the switch to cyclosporine therapy. Another liver biopsy was performed which indicated the presence of recurrent HCV disease. The patient was treated again with Rebetron and a subsequent liver biopsy at year 2 as shown in Figure 4-6 demonstrated resolution of the recurrent HCV infection.

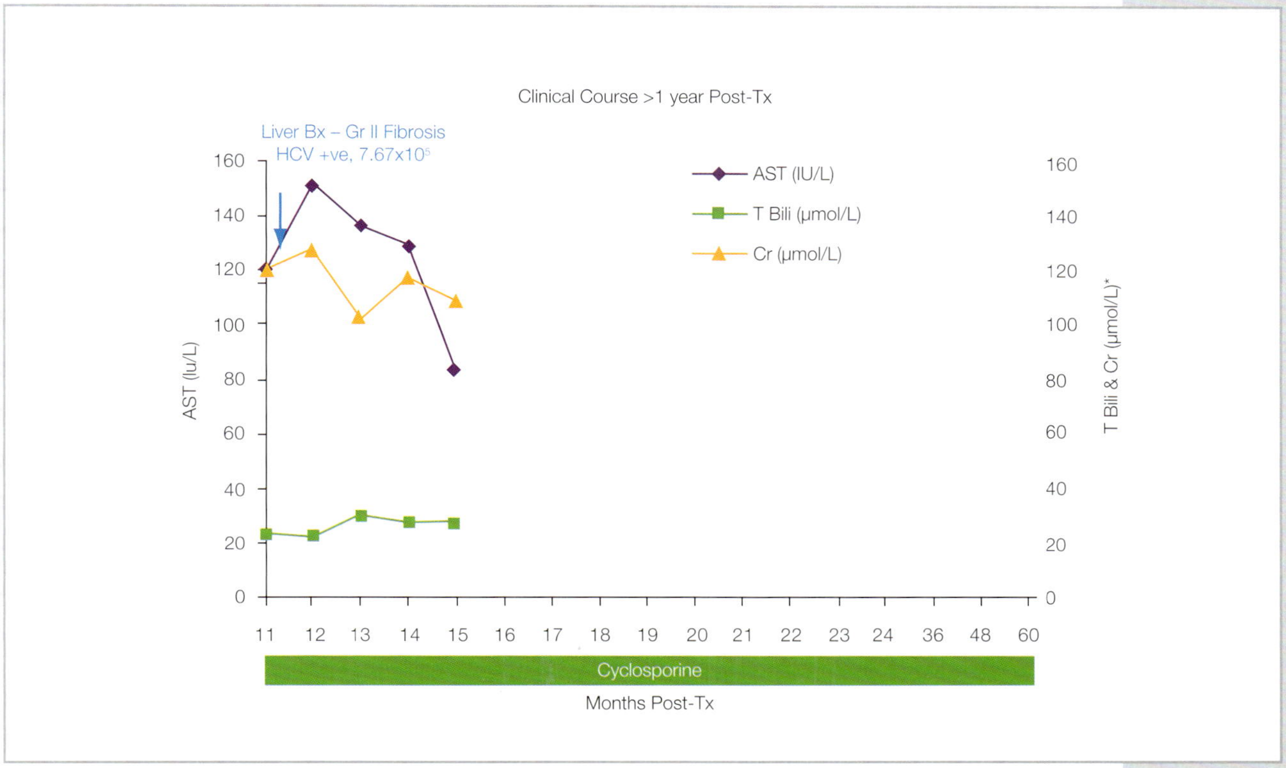

* Creatinine 1 mg/dL = 88.4 μmol/L; Bilirubin 1 mg/dL = 17.1 μmol/L

FIGURE 4-5. Clinical course of the liver transplant recipient during cyclosporine immunosuppressive therapy.

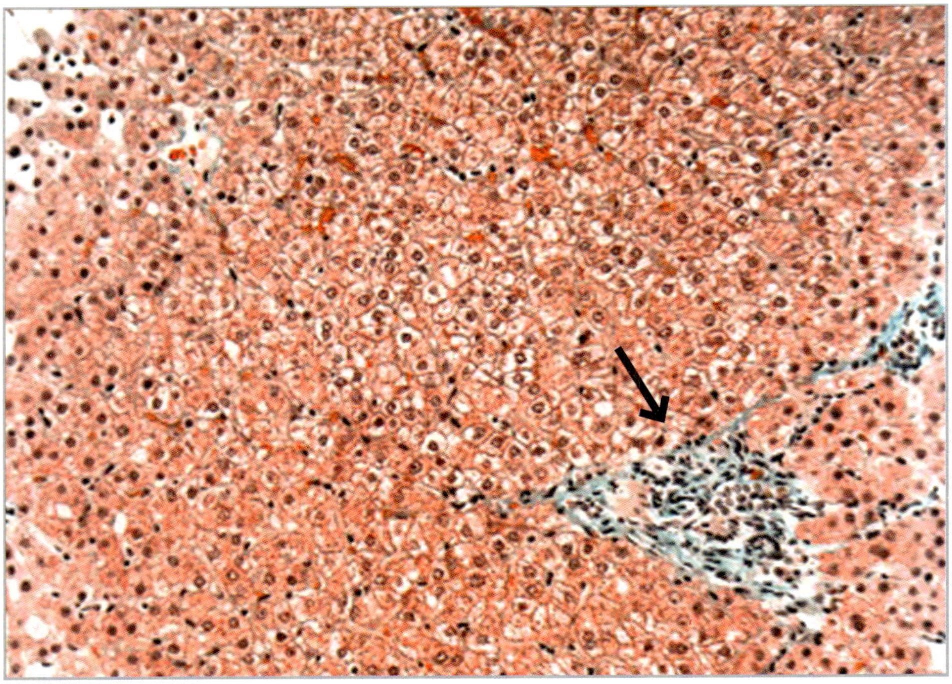

FIGURE 4-6. Trichrome stain of liver biopsy post-Rebetron therapy showing normal portal triad (arrow) and hepatic architecture (magnification x200).

CASE HISTORY 3: LIVER TRANSPLANT RECIPIENT WITH RECURRENT HCV INFECTION

Patient with cirrhosis of the liver caused by chronic HCV infection

A 51 year-old man was referred for liver transplantation. He was suffering from cirrhosis caused by chronic hepatitis C. He acquired hepatitis C as a result of factor infusions required for treatment of hemophilia A. He was diagnosed with hepatitis C 17 years earlier and was treated with non-PEG-interferon 11 years ago for 1 year without response.

Clinical and Medical History

- Hemophilia A, treated for >40 years with factor transfusions.
- Chronic HCV infection.
- Cirrhosis for 2 years.
- Variceal bleeding controlled by sclerotherapy.
- Ascites, encephalopathy at best modestly controlled by medical therapy yielding poor quality of life.
- HIV positive, managed with Truvada and a protease inhibitor.
- HIV RNA (-).
- CD4 426 cell/mm^3.
- No opportunistic infections.
- Insulin-dependent diabetes.
- Multiple joint bleeds.
- No alcohol or tobacco use.
- Two brothers with hemophilia, one who died of HIV, the other is well.

Physical Exam

- Remarkable for no scleral icterus.
- Muscle atrophy.
- Ascites.
- Hyperpigmentation over lower extremities.
- Multiple joint deformities.

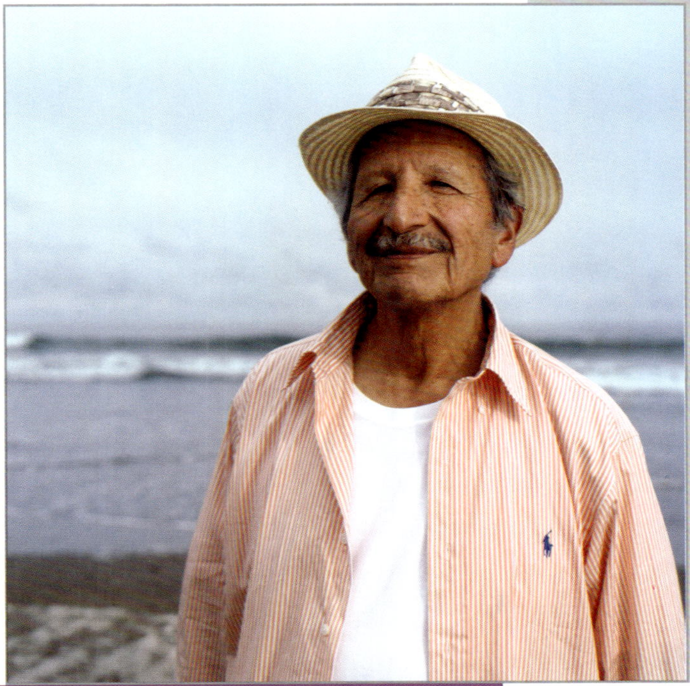

Pre-Transplant Laboratory Findings

- AST of 43 IU/L.
- ALT of 42 IU/L.
- Bilirubin 2.9 mg/dL (49.6 µmol/L).
- Albumin 26 g/L (2.6 g/dL).
- Serum creatinine 1.9 mg/dL (168.0 µmol/L).
- Prothrombin time 1.8 INR.
- HCV positive, genotype 1A virus.
- HCV viral load 6.3 log IU/mL.

Clinical and laboratory findings indicate a liver transplant was the appropriate therapy.

Liver transplantation

Orthotopic liver transplantation (OLT) was performed without difficulty with the biliary reconstruction consisting of a choledocho-choledochostomy. An incidental, 3 cm hepatocellular carcinoma was found on examination of the explant.

Immunosuppressive Therapy

- Tacrolimus
- MMF
- Corticosteroids

Day 7 Post-transplant Laboratory Results

- Immediate allograft function.
- AST 40 IU/L.
- Alkaline phosphatase 138 IU/L.
- Bilirubin 6.2 mg/dL (106.0 µmol/L).

Day 12 Hospital Discharge

- Oral tacrolimus, prednisone, MMF.
- Liver tests excellent.
- AST 18 IU/L.
- Alkaline phosphatase 96 IU/L.
- Bilirubin 2.0 mg/dL (34.2 µmol/L).
- Serum creatinine 2.2 mg/dL (194.5 µmol/L).
- Oral tacrolimus dose reduced 50%.

Day 19 Liver Test Values Elevated

- AST 296 IU/L.
- Alkaline phosphatase 497 IU/L.
- Bilirubin 7.0 mg/dL (119.7 µmol/L).
- Liver biopsy performed.

Liver Biopsy Result

The biopsy showed acute cellular rejection (see Figures 4-7 and 4-8). In general, this is treated with additional immunosuppression either in the form of corticosteroid boluses or in some cases anti-lymphocyte antibody therapy. Treated rejection has been associated with worse outcomes in patients transplanted for hepatitis C so one should always treat rejection with caution in such patients. In some cases one might first try to simply maximize the maintenance immunosuppressive drug concentration.

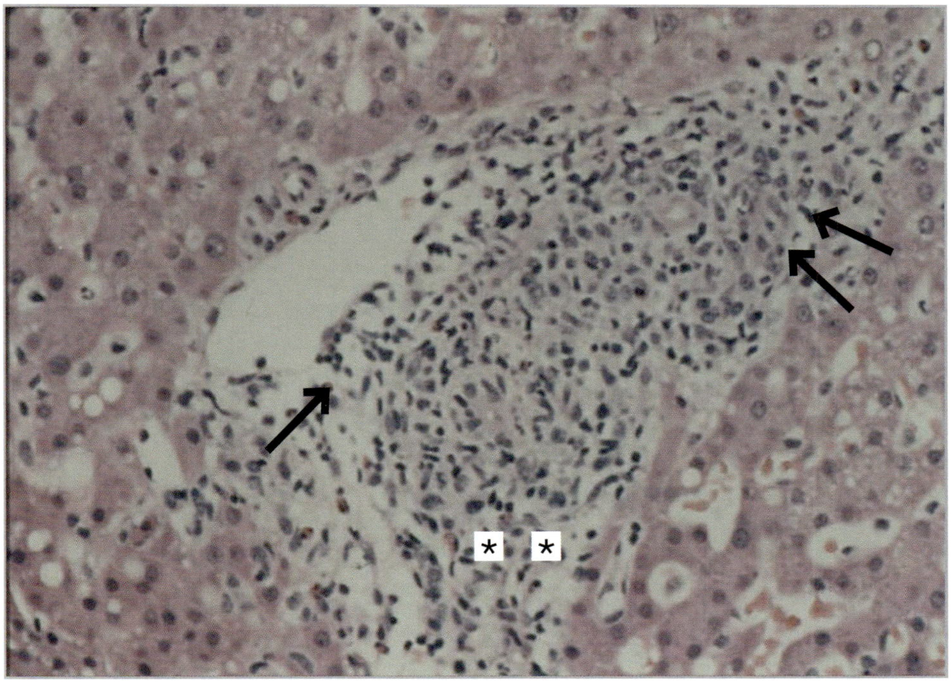

FIGURE 4-7. Liver biopsy showing acute cellular rejection characterized by portal vein inflammation (vasculitis) and eosinophils (asterisk) with bile duct injury (arrow).

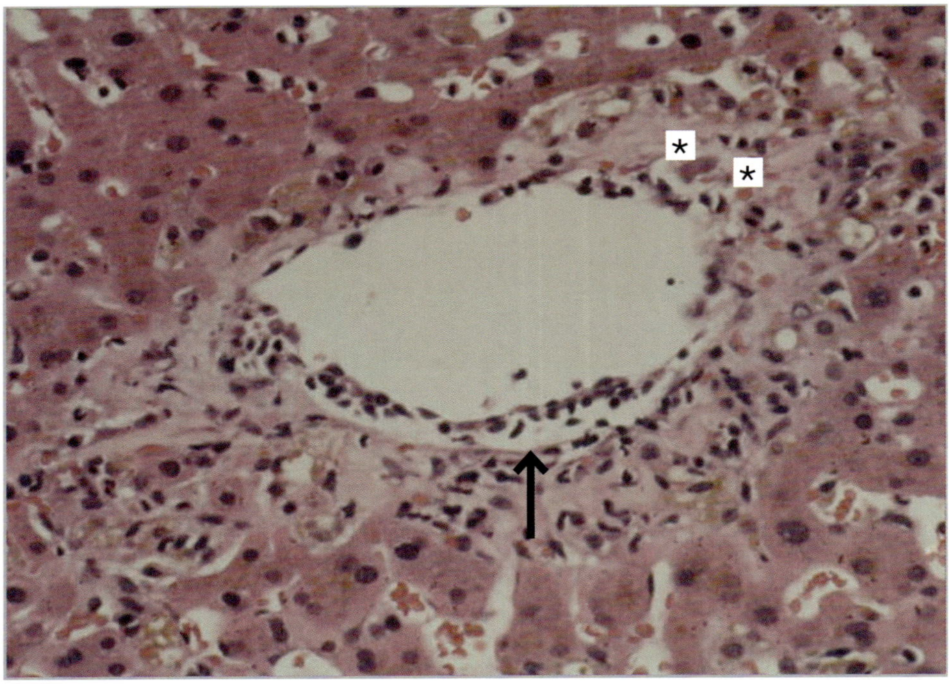

FIGURE 4-8. Liver biopsy showing improvement in rejection, but still showing portal vein vasculitis (arrow) and the presence of eosinophils (asterisk).

Patient Follow-up for Rejection

- Two 1 gram methylprednisolone boluses.
- Prednisone recycle.
- Follow-up liver biopsy 2 weeks later.
- Biopsy showed mild fatty change but no rejection.
- AST 15 IU/L.
- Alkaline phosphatase 245 IU/L.
- Bilirubin 1.6 mg/dL (27.4 µmol/L).
- Tacrolimus 16 ng/mL.

Patient Follow-up 1 Month Later

- AST 155 IU/L (elevated).
- Alkaline phosphatase 178 IU/L (unchanged).
- Liver biopsy performed.

Second Liver Biopsy Result

The second liver biopsy, shown in Figure 4-9, showed hepatocyte necrosis and mild portal inflammation consistent with post-transplant hepatitis or resolving rejection. The clinical impression was that the findings were due to recurrent hepatitis C infection and tacrolimus and prednisone were continued, but MMF was discontinued. Over the next month, the liver tests improved. Recurrent hepatitis C can be difficult to differentiate from acute rejection. For the reasons mentioned earlier, one does not want to over treat rejection in these patients.

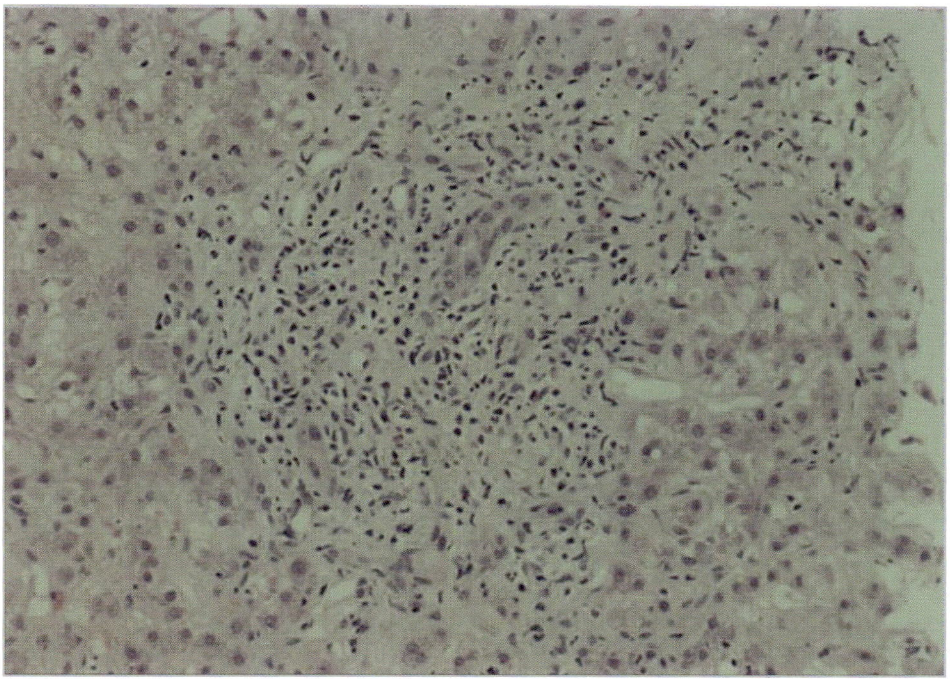

FIGURE 4-9. Second liver biopsy result showing post-transplant hepatitis or resolving rejection.

At one year post-OLT, a protocol liver biopsy was also performed.

Protocol Liver Biopsy Result at 1 Year Post-transplant

This showed the typical appearance of recurrent hepatitis C infection as shown in Figure 4-10. The main question at this point would be whether to treat the recurrence of hepatitis C infection.

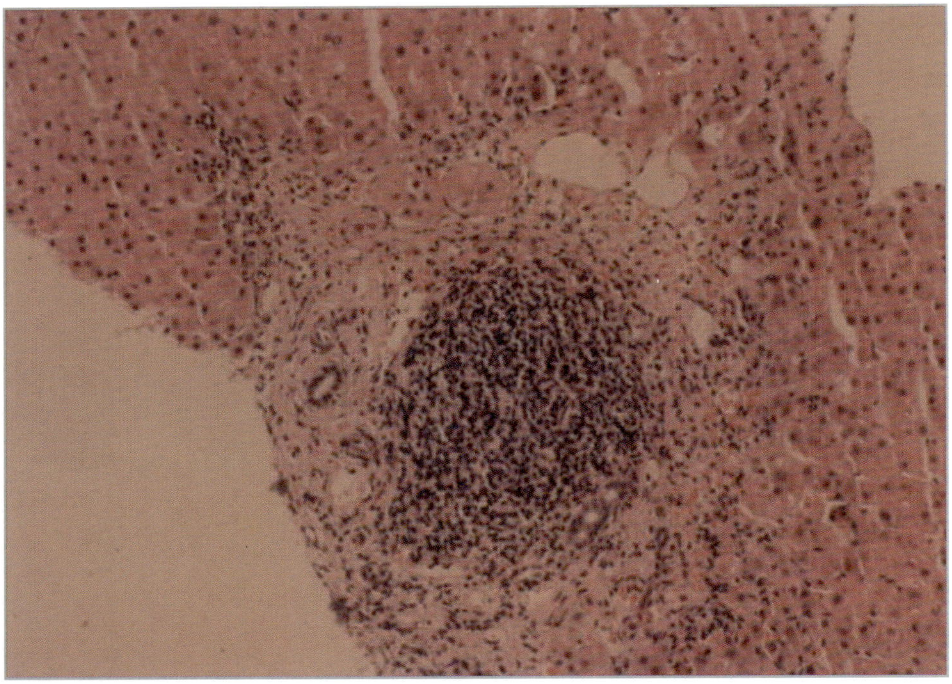

FIGURE 4-10. Recurrent HCV infection at one year post-transplant.

CASE HISTORY 4: THE IMPACT OF BK VIRUS INFECTION FOLLOWING RENAL TRANSPLANTATION

Patient with Chronic Renal Failure who Received a Kidney Allograft

A 45-year-old diabetic man with chronic renal failure received a non-HLA matched kidney transplant from a deceased donor. The patient had a 15-year history of type 2 diabetes mellitus. The allograft was considered an expanded criteria donor kidney because the donor's age was 61 years. Cold ischemic time was 17 hours and warm ischemic time was 55 minutes. Both donor and recipient were CMV and EBV positive. Serum creatinine at transplant was 6.8 mg/dL (601.1 µmol/L).

Immunosuppressive Therapy

- Induction therapy, 20 mg basiliximab.
- Cyclosporine, oral.
- MMF, oral.
- Prednisone, oral.

The patient experienced post-operative atrial fibrillation and atrial flutter for which he was treated with amiodarone hydrochloride at an initial dose of 200 mg orally qd (once daily) and warfarin sodium 5 mg orally qd.

Early Post-operative Period

- Day 3
  Marginal graft function, serum creatinine 6.0 mg/dL (530.4 µmol/L).
  Good urine output, no dialysis required.
- Day 4
  20 mg basiliximab.
  Cyclosporine target range 250 to 300 ng/mL, months 1-3, 12-hour trough concentration.
  MMF 1 g bid.
  Steroid taper.
- Day 10
  Serum creatinine 2.2 mg/dL (194.5 µmol/L).
  Renal function monitored every 3 to 7 days during weeks 4 through 12.
  At 4 weeks serum creatinine was 1.8 mg/dL (159.1 µmol/L).

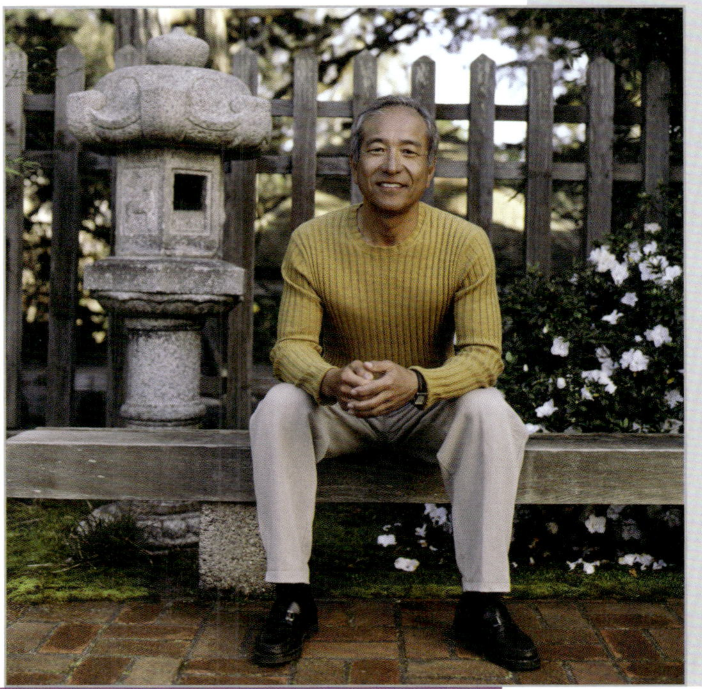

Five Weeks Post-transplant: Impaired Graft Function with BK Viral Infection

Five weeks after transplantation, a sample of the patient's urine was sent for cytologic examination because of ongoing impaired graft function, i.e. elevated serum creatinine of 1.9 mg/dL (168.0 µmol/L), and because he was known to have multiple risk factors for BK virus-associated nephropathy.

The urine sample showed cytologic changes consistent with BK viral infection, which was confirmed by immunostaining as shown in Figure 4-11. At that time, the patient's medications were cyclosporine 150 mg orally bid, MMF 1 g orally bid, and prednisone 20 mg orally qd. The presence of BK virus nephropathy should mandate a lowering of immunosuppression. The patient's cyclosporine blood concentration was 238 ng/mL when the decoy cells were detected.

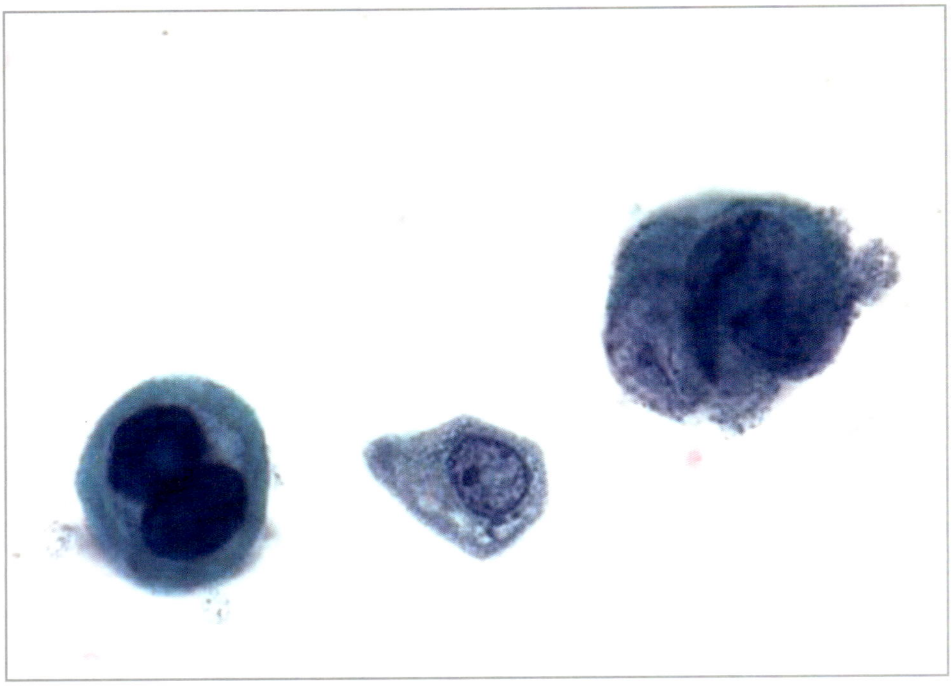

FIGURE 4-11. Immunostain showing BK virus nephropathy as indicated by typical decoy cells in urine.

Eight Weeks Post-transplant: Rising Serum Creatinine

- Serum creatinine 2.6 mg/dL (229.8 μmol/L).
- Kidney biopsy performed.
- BK viral inclusions in tubular and glomerular epithelial cells.
- Diagnosis of BK virus infection reinforced.

Immunosuppressive Therapy Changes

- Switch from cyclosporine to 5 mg sirolimus qd.
- Taper cyclosporine over 5 days.
- Sirolimus dose adjusted to maintain target concentrations of 10-12 ng/mL.
- MMF decreased to 750 mg bid per routine taper.
- Prednisone decreased to 10 mg orally qd.

Less than 1 month after the patient's treatment was switched from cyclosporine to sirolimus, the patient's urine cytology was negative for BK polyoma virus effect. His serum creatinine had stabilized in the range of 1.8-2.1 mg/dL (159.1-185.6 μmol/L).

Nine months Post-transplant: Normal Renal Function, No Decoy Cells

- Serum creatinine 1.9 mg/dL (168.0 μmol/L).
- No decoy cell shedding in the urine.

Maintenance Immunosuppressive Regimen

- Sirolimus 2 mg orally qd.
- MMF 250 mg orally bid.
- Prednisone 4 mg orally qd.

Renal function was monitored monthly. Laboratory workups, including monitoring sirolimus concentration and urine cytologic examinations to screen for the presence of decoy cells, were performed every 3 months.

05 FUTURE OF SOLID ORGAN TRANSPLANTATION AND THERAPEUTIC DRUG MONITORING

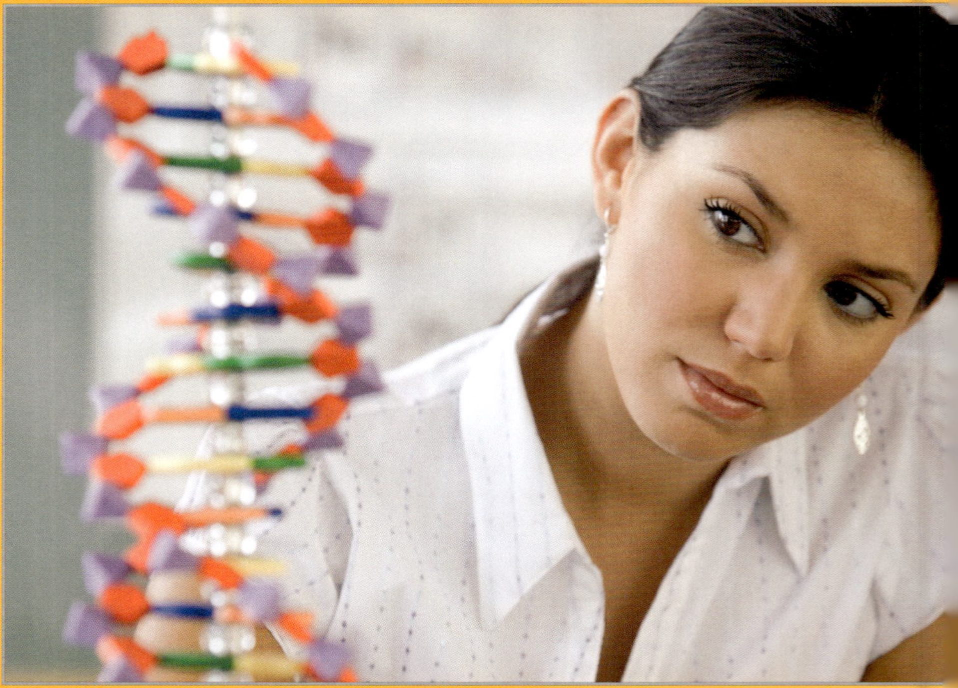

CHAPTER 5 CONTENTS

DRUG MINIMIZATION

The present use of immunosuppressants is associated with organ specific or systemic toxicities. Among the major agents being used today, the calcineurin inhibitors tacrolimus and cyclosporine and corticosteroids are associated with clinically relevant undesired adverse effects. These adverse effects lead to damage of transplanted organs and accelerate development of diabetes and cardiovascular disease, which shorten patients' lives. In an effort to minimize or avoid toxicity and to improve patient quality of life, efforts are now underway towards avoiding, withdrawing, or minimizing exposure to these agents.

CORTICOSTEROID WITHDRAWAL

The morbidities associated with the use of corticosteroids are well documented and can be substantial, as shown in Table 5-1.

TABLE 5-1. Long-Term Corticosteroid Morbidities

Glucose Intolerance	Dyslipidemia
Hypertension	Osteoporosis
Infection	Cataracts
Dermal Atrophy	Weight Gain

Success in reducing or eliminating corticosteroids has been limited by the risk of acute rejection and the development of late allograft loss. Initial reports suggested that, although corticosteroids could be withdrawn, renal transplant patients on steroid-free regimens had a high incidence of chronic allograft nephropathy leading to graft loss. More recently, steroid reduction and withdrawal has been performed safely in both renal and liver transplant patients, although the incidence of acute rejection is higher in patients on steroid-free protocols and withdrawal is associated with acute rejection. The introduction of MMF has now allowed early discontinuation of steroids, with a reduction in adverse effects, including improvement in glucose homeostasis, lipid profiles and improvement in blood pressure, without loss of graft function at 5 years post steroid discontinuation. Based on a number of large multi-center trials, steroid avoidance protocols or withdrawal of corticosteroids as early as 1 week post transplant, is becoming standard practice in many centers. Early steroid withdrawal does not impact negatively on patient or graft survival in kidney transplantation. A summary of benefits and risks of early corticosteroid withdrawal (CSWD) relative to chronic low dose corticosteroid therapy (CCS) in renal allograft recipients is shown in Table 5-2. A comparison of four different immunosuppressive drug regimens without long-term corticosteroid therapy in kidney transplant recipients is shown in Figure 5-1.

TABLE 5-2. Summary of Benefits and Risks of Early CSWD

Benefits: Secondary Endpoints	Time point (Mo)	Statistical Parameter (Test Used)	P	Group Favored
Triglycerides* (all)	48	Mean; t test	0.001	CSWD
Triglycerides* (patients w/o hyperlipidemia at enrollment)	60	Mean; t test	0.004	CSWD
Serum cholesterol*	48	Mean; t test	0.081	CSWD
Hyperlipidemia therapy (all)	60	Proportion; Fisher exact	0.053	CSWD
Hyperlipidemia therapy (patients w/o hyperlipidemia at enrollment)	60	Proportion; Fisher exact	0.038	CSWD
Weight gain*	60	Median; Wilcoxon	0.05	CSWD
NODAT requiring insulin	60	Proportion; Fisher exact	0.049	CSWD
HgA1c* (patients w/o pre-Tx diabetes)	48	Mean; t test	0.039	CSWD
HgA1c* (patients with new onset post-Tx diabetes)	60	Mean; t test	0.048	CSWD
Benefits: Post-hoc analyses	**Time point (Mo)**	**Statistical Parameter (Test Used)**	**P**	**Group Favored**
Avascular necrosis	60	Proportion; Fisher exact	0.061	CSWD
Avascular necrosis or fractures	60	Proportion; Fisher exact	0.041	CSWD
Hospitalized patients	60	Proportion; Fisher exact	0.065	CSWD
Risks: Secondary Endpoints	**Time point (Mo)**	**Statistical Parameter (Test Used)**	**P**	**Group Favored**
Biopsy confirmed acute rejection	60	Kaplan Meier; log rank	0.042	CCS
Chronic allograft nephropathy	60	Proportion; Fisher exact	0.028	CCS

*Evaluated change from pre-transplant
Statistically significant difference (P value <0.05); trend, P value >0.05, <0.09.
Adapted from Woodle et al. (2008).

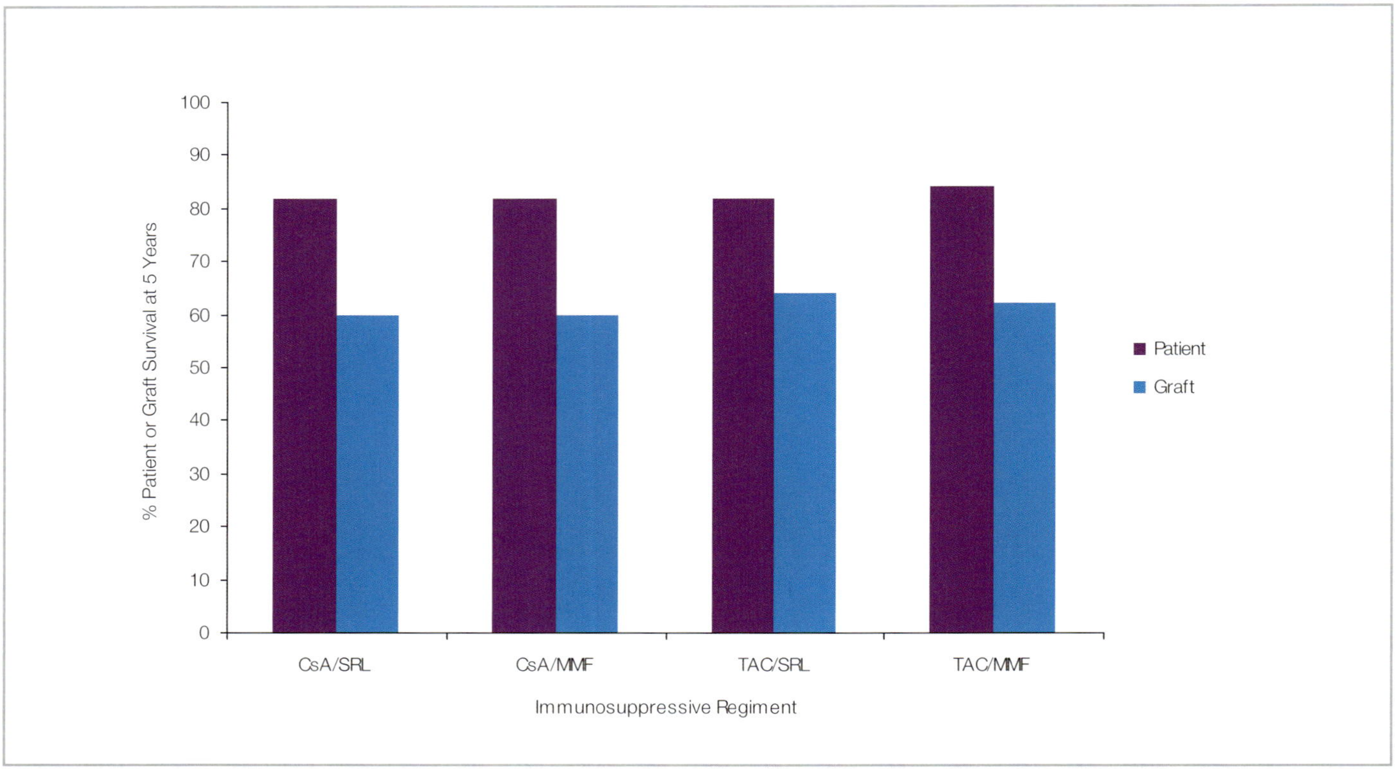

FIGURE 5-1. Comparison of four different immunosuppressive regimens without long-term corticosteroid therapy: Patient and graft survival rates in kidney recipients treated with CsA/MMF, CsA/SRL, TAC/MMF, and TAC/SRL immunosuppression therapy. CsA, cyclosporine; MMF, Mycophenolate mofetil,; SRL, Sirolimus; TAC, Tacrolimus. Adapted from Kumar (2008).

CNI WITHDRAWAL/MINIMIZATION

The primary impetus to reduce or eliminate CNIs in transplant patients has resulted from concerns about their known adverse effects including the development of diabetes, accelerated atherosclerosis, hypertension, heart disease and nephrotoxicity. This is balanced by the observation that the use of CNIs has led to a marked improvement in short-term patient and graft survival. Furthermore, although use of CNIs is associated with fibrointimal changes in the vasculature and fibrotic atrophic changes in the tubulointerstitial compartment, it is not totally clear whether these changes are due to the use of CNIs or as a result of alloimmune injury. In fact a recent study by Nankivall (2004) has suggested that the major risk factor for the development of chronic renal injury in renal transplant patients is low concentrations of tacrolimus and a high incidence of acute rejection. The development of newer agents, including the mTOR inhibitors sirolimus and everolimus and the nucleotide synthesis inhibitor MMF, may allow safe reduction of CNI without the risk of rejection. Results from the large European multi-centered ELITE-Symphony trial, as discussed earlier in this monograph, have shown that treating patients with reduced levels of tacrolimus or cyclosporine in combination with MMF and steroids can lead to improved renal function and a reduction in the incidence of hypertension, hyperlipidemia and diabetes mellitus in comparison to patients on standard immunosuppression. Weir et al. (2004) have reported that cyclosporine withdrawal in patients with deteriorating graft function can lead to stabilization or even improvement in renal function. Pascual and co-workers (2008) have reported recently that treatment with a CNI avoidance protocol comprising Campath, sirolimus, and MMF can be used successfully in renal transplant patients, whereas a protocol of sirolimus, MMF and corticosteroids did not appear to have advantages for long-term graft function. In another review by Srinivas and co-workers (2007), sirolimus/MMF was associated with poorer renal transplant outcomes when compared to other common immunosuppressive regimens. A summary of CNI-minimization or withdrawal studies in transplant recipients with stable renal function is shown in Table 5-3.

In addition to studying different combinations of drugs, new immunosuppressive agents being assessed for utility include Belatacept, a co-stimulation inhibitor, a JAK 3 kinase anti-proliferative inhibitor, and AEB071, a protein kinase C inhibitor that blocks T cell activation through a CNI-independent pathway (see Chapter 2, Figure 2-5 for sites of action). If their efficacy and safety are established, randomized trials will be performed to optimize their use in different immunosuppressive cocktails.

TABLE 5-3. CNI-minimization or Withdrawal in Recipients with Stable Renal Function

IS Therapy withdrawal vs. control	Time of IS change post-Tx	AR rates withdrawal vs. control	Renal function change vs. control	Follow-up
MMF-Pred vs. AZA-Pred	12 mo	11.8% vs. 36.7% (p<0.05)	Improved from baseline in both arms	20 mo
MMF-Pred vs. CsA-MMF-Pred	6 mo	22% vs. 1.4% (p<0.05)	Improved	24 mo
MMF-Pred vs. CsA-MMF-Pred	12-30 mo	9.5% vs. 1.3% (p<0.05)	Improved	5 yr
MMF-Pred vs. CsA-Pred	3 mo	11.3% vs. 5.0% (NS)	Improved	12 mo
50%CsA-Pred vs. CsA-Pred	>12 mo	No rejection	Improved	6 mo
MMF-Pred vs. Low-CsA-MMF-Pred vs. CsA-MMF-Pred (CAESAR)	6 mo	38% vs. 25.4% vs. 27.5% (p<0.05)	No difference	12 mo
SRL-Pred vs. CsA-SRL-Pred (RMR)	3 mo	10.2% vs. 6.5% (NS)	Improved	48 mo
SRL-MMF-Pred vs. CNI-MMF-Pred (Spare-The-Nephron)	30-180 d	6.5% vs. 7.1% (NS)	Improved	12 mo

AR, acute rejection; AZA, azathioprine; CNI, calcineurin inhibitors; CsA, cyclosporine; IS, immunosuppression; mo, months; yr, year, d, day; MMF, Mycophenolate mofetil; NS, non-significant; Pred, prednisone; SRL, sirolimus; TAC, tacrolimus; Tx, transplantation
Adapted from Golshayan (2008).

FUTURE APPROACHES TO TDM

Therapeutic drug monitoring of immunosuppressive drugs remains a major support for the management of transplant patients. It can assist the clinician in patient management by highlighting poor compliance, identifying drug interactions, and providing information on actual drug exposure. Further progress and contributions of TDM should be focused on patient quality of life and personalized immunosuppression.

There is strong evidence for a relationship between drug exposure and patient outcomes (adverse effects and treatment efficacy). The routine determination of a drug concentration at C_0 is used to assess drug exposure, even though it might not be the optimal marker of either exposure or efficacy. Progress still needs to be made to improve the prediction of efficacy and may result from the following research areas:

- Since AUC is unanimously considered a better marker of exposure, improvement of predictive value could be obtained through the help of population pharmacokinetic models with Bayesian estimators and multi-center validation.
- Drug concentrations at the target sites (e.g. lymphocytes) should be more relevant than whole blood drug concentrations, in predicting treatment efficacy. An understanding of all the factors influencing drug concentrations at the target sites could help to improve the prediction of efficacy.
- Pharmacogenetics may contribute to a better understanding of drug disposition in an individual patient. This could facilitate attaining adequate blood concentrations more predictably and, hopefully, adequate drug concentration at target sites.
- There is clearly a trend to consider pharmacodynamic biomarkers, for example, cytokines as complementary promising biomarkers. Progress in defining the best pharmacodynamic biomarkers as well as in standardizing their measurement should contribute substantially to improving the monitoring of transplant patients.
- Lower dose therapies will require clinical laboratories to use TDM assays with good low end precision and high functional sensitivity in order to measure reliably the lower drug concentrations present in these transplant recipients.

The progress in these different research areas, together with further analytical improvements in the measurement of the drugs (specificity, sensitivity, precision and robustness) will draw and define the future of TDM in transplantation.

FUTURE APPROACHES TO IMMUNE MONITORING AND INFLAMMATION

Currently, transplant patients are monitored for freedom from rejection using assays that measure blood concentrations of immune suppressants. Clearly, although helpful, they have not proven to be totally reliable and, despite adequate therapeutic concentrations, many patients develop acute or chronic allograft rejection. Furthermore, these assays have not prevented long term drug toxicity, infections, or development of cancers, which are known complications of their use. A number of new biologic assays have appeared, with the potential to act as markers of inflammation or to predict the immune status of the host.

THE IMMUKNOW ASSAY

The ImmuKnow® assay is a biologic test that measures ATP production by CD4+ T cells to broad stimulation by the lectin phytohemagglutinin (PHA). Low concentrations < 200 ng/mL have been reported to be associated with over immunosuppression and the risk of developing life threatening infections. Concentrations > 450 ng/mL were associated with under immunosuppression and a higher risk of rejection, as shown in Figure 5-2. Studies are now underway to assess the utility of this assay in transplant patients.

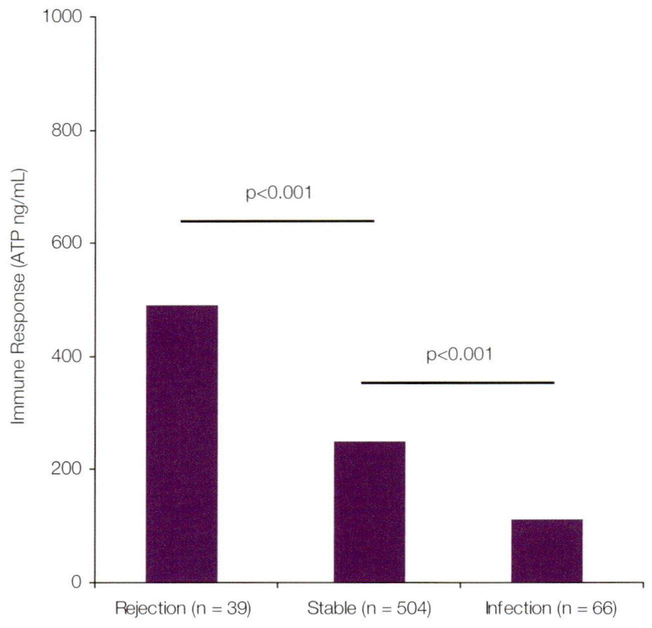

FIGURE 5-2. Immune response during periods of rejection, stability, and infection in solid organ transplant recipients. Adapted from Kowalski et al. (2006).

NEUTROPHIL GELATINASE–ASSOCIATED LIPOCALIN (NGAL)

Lipocalin (NGAL) is a 25 kDa protein produced by neutrophils. It is elevated in the serum of patients with bacterial infection, asthma, or chronic obstructive pulmonary disease (COPD). Elevated levels of NGAL have been observed in the blood and urine of patients with renal disease. NGAL levels appear to correlate with serum creatinine and these levels have been found to be a powerful independent predictor of acute kidney injury. In renal transplantation Parikh and co-workers (2008) have found that urinary NGAL measured on Day 0 of deceased donor kidney transplantation predicts delayed graft function earlier than other clinical markers currently in use (see Figure 5-3).

It remains unclear whether we can use NGAL to monitor graft function, differentiate rejection from chronic allograft nephropathy (CAN), or use NGAL to differentiate pre-renal from hepatorenal syndrome and/or CNI toxicity.

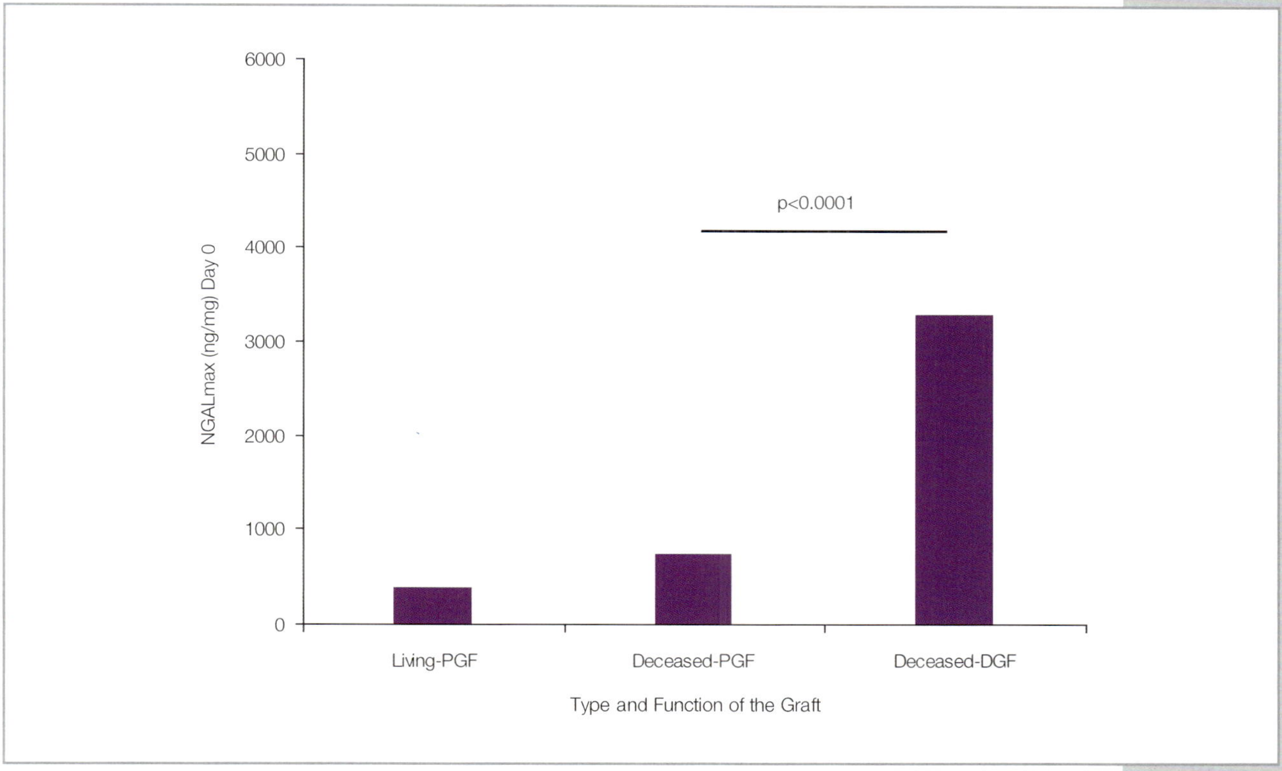

FIGURE 5-3. Urinary NGAL levels in the first 24 hours after renal transplantation.

Living-PGF: Living donor, prompt graft function.
Deceased-PGF: Deceased donor, prompt graft function.
Deceased-DGF: Deceased donor, delayed graft function.
Adapted from Parikh et al. (2006).

GENOMICS/PROTEOMICS

The availability of microarray technology for genome-wide transcriptosome analysis potentially offers the hope for objective and quantitative diagnosis and insights into the pathogenesis of allograft rejection. Furthermore, this technology may allow us to predict which patients have developed tolerance. A number of reports have emerged that identify gene markers associated with allograft rejection, ischemia reperfusion injury, early graft function and, most recently, potential gene markers for tolerance. Figure 5-4 describes the process of gene expression profiling in transplant recipients.

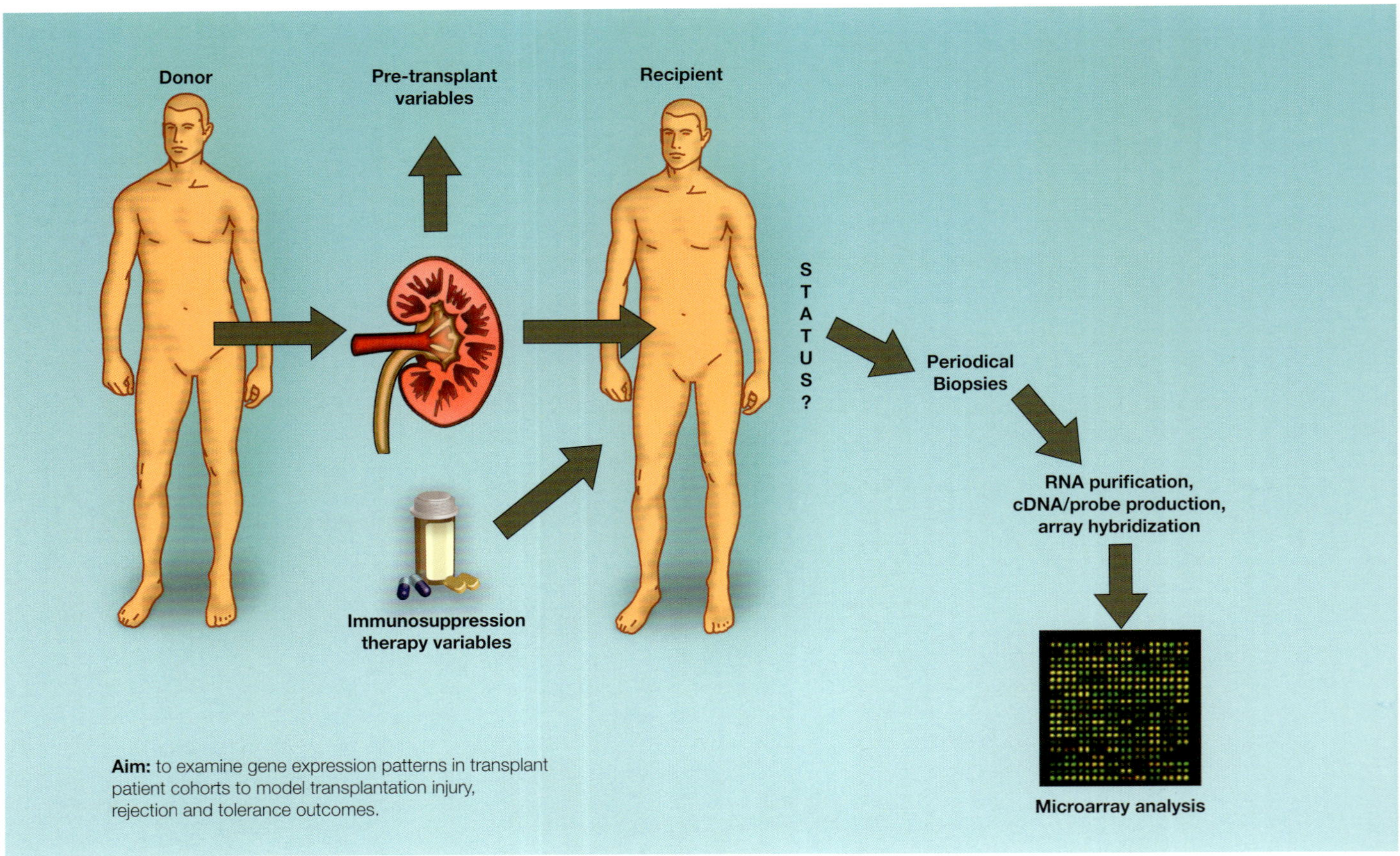

FIGURE 5-4. Gene expression profiling in transplant recipients.

Data from these and other studies have suggested that the presence of $CD4^+CD25^+FoxP3^+$ T regulatory cells (Treg) in the allograft may reflect a state of tolerance, although in some reports the presence of these cells may reflect an attempt to control inflammation. Other investigators have now begun to look at the proteome and metabolome in an attempt to define tolerance and/or mechanisms of graft injury. The Levy research group has established a highly reproducible ELISA to measure an effector cytokine of Treg and preliminary data, shown in Figure 5-5, suggest that levels of the cytokine FGL2/fibroleukin may predict a state of immunologic tolerance (graft acceptance without the need for long-term immunosuppression) and allow for reduction/elimination of immunosuppression. A prospective trial is now underway to examine this hypothesis.

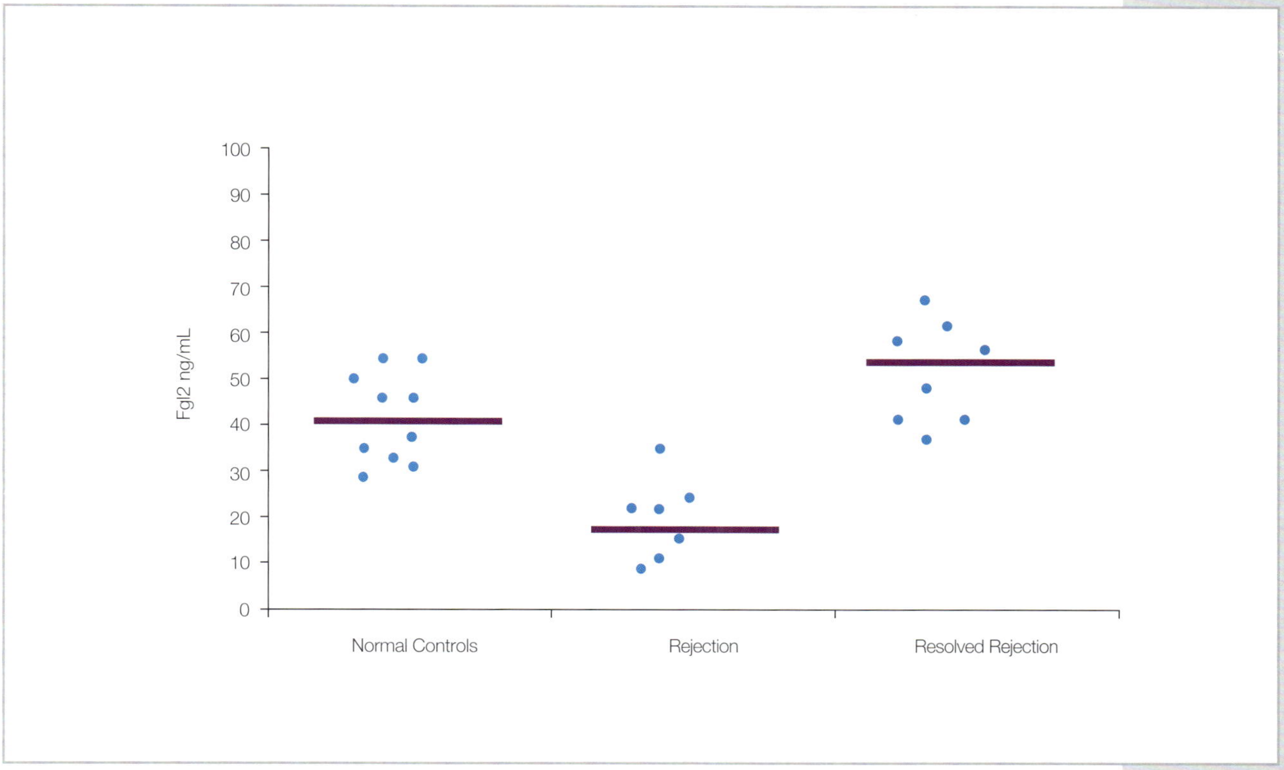

FIGURE 5-5. Fgl2 and transplantation.

KEY QUESTIONS FOR THE FUTURE OF SOLID ORGAN TRANSPLANTATION AND TDM

- Can we adopt better assays (AUC, C_2) to monitor immunosuppressive agents?
- Will biologic assays (ImmuKnow, NGAL) augment or replace present assays to monitor immune status of the patient?
- Will genomic monitoring identify specific markers for tolerance/rejection?

BIBLIOGRAPHY FOR CHAPTER 5

Golshayan D and Pascual M. Minimization of calcineurin inhibitors to improve long-term outcomes in kidney transplantation. Transplant Immunol. 2008;20:21-8.

Woodle ES, First MR, Pirsch J et al. A prospective, randomized, double-blind, placebo-controlled multicenter trial comparing early (7 day) corticosteroid cessation versus long-term, low-dose corticosteroid therapy. Annals of Surgery. 2008;248:564-77.

Sayegh MH, Carpenter CB. Transplantation 50 years later-progress, challenges, and promises. N Engl J Med. 2004;351:2761-6.

Flechner SM, Kobashigawa J, Klintmalm G. Calcineurin inhibitor sparing regimens in solid organ transplantation: Focus on improving renal function and nephrotoxicity. Clin Transplant. 2008;22:1-15.

Kumar MSA, Saeed MI, Ranganna K et al. Comparison of four different immunosuppression protocols without long-term steroid therapy in kidney recipients monitored by surveillance biopsy: Five-year outcomes. Transplant Immunol. 2008;20:32-42.

Parikh CR, Jani A, Mishra J et al. Urine NGAL and IL-18 are predictive biomarkers for delayed graft function following kidney transplantation. Amer J Transplant. 2006;6:1639-45.

Sarwal M, Chua MS, Kambham N et al. Molecular heterogeneity in acute renal allograft rejection identified by DNA microarray profiling. N Engl J Med. 2003;349:125-38.

Liu H, Shalev I, Manuel J, He W, Leung E, Crookshank J, Liu MF et al. The Fgl2-FcGRIIB pathway: a novel mechanism leading to immunosuppression. Euro J Immunol. 2008;38:3114-26.

Nankivell BJ, Borrows RJ, Fung CLS et al. Evolution and pathophysiology of renal-transplant glomulerosclerosis. Transplantation. 2004;78:461-8.

Kowalski RJ, Post DR, Mannon RB et al. Assessing relative risks of infection and rejection: A meta-analysis using an immune function assay. Transplantation 2006;82:663-8.

Weir MR, Blahut S, Drachenburg C et al. Late calcineurin inhibitor withdrawal as a strategy to prevent graft loss in patients with suboptimal kidney transplant function. Amer J Nephro. 2004;24:379-86.

Pascual J, Bloom D, Torrealba J et al. Calcineurin inhibitor withdrawal after renal transplantation with alemtuzumab: clinical outcomes and effect on regulatory T-cells. Amer J Transplant. 2008;8:1529-36.

Srinivas TR, Schold JD, Guerra G et al. Mycophenolate mofetil/sirolimus compared to other common immunosuppressive regimens in kidney transplantation. Amer J Transplant. 2007;7:586-94.

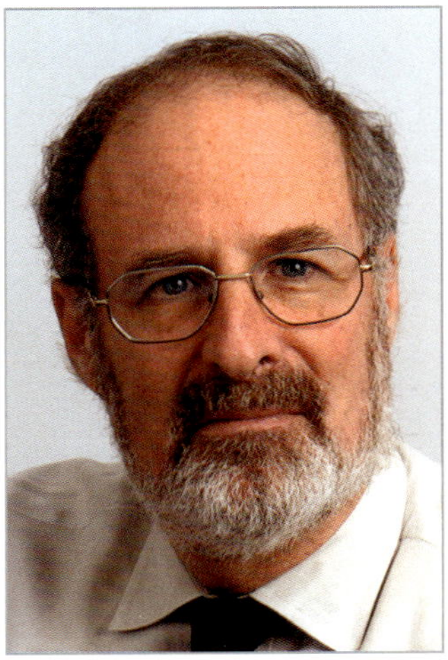

Gary A. Levy, MD

Professor of Medicine, University of Toronto
Director, Multi Organ Transplant Program
University Health Network – University of Toronto

Dr. Levy graduated from medical school at the University of Toronto in 1973. He completed his training in hepatology at the University of Toronto in 1978 and undertook postdoctoral training in immunology at the Scripps Clinic and Research Foundation from 1978-81. Dr. Levy founded and became the Medical Director of the Liver Transplant Unit at the Toronto General Hospital and University of Toronto in 1987. In 1991, he organized and co-founded their Multi Organ Transplant Unit.

He is currently a Professor in the Departments of Medicine and Surgery at the University of Toronto and Director of the Multi Organ Transplant Program at the University Health Network and University of Toronto.

He has organized and now heads a research group of 11 principle investigators which is focused on studying cellular and molecular mechanisms of inflammation. His research has continuously been funded by the Canadian Institutes for Health Research for over 25 years, the National Institutes of Health, and the Heart and Stroke Foundation of Canada and has focused on immune-mediated mechanisms of organ injury due to viruses, alloantigens, and xenoantigens. He is the Director of the CIHR Training Program in Regenerative Medicine and was recently awarded 20 million dollars from the Canada Foundation for Innovation to build research capacity for studies on immune tolerance. He has published over 318 original articles, books and book chapters. He currently holds the Novartis Chair in Transplantation at the University of Toronto.

He has received a number of honors including election to the American Society for Clinical Investigation, the Goldie Prize in Medicine, the Canadian Association of Gastroenterology Visiting Research Professorship and the University of Toronto, Department of Medicine Research Award for outstanding contributions to research. He has been an Honorary Professor of Tongi Medical College of Huazhong University of Science and Technology since October 2001. He is a member of the following editorial boards: Transplantation Science, Transplantation, Transplant Proceedings and Current Opinion in Organ Transplantation and is a member of an advisory board for Health Canada in transplantation and xenotransplantation. He served as the Chief Scientific Officer of Transplantation Technologies Inc., from 1997 to 2002. He was the President of the Canadian Digestive Health Foundation from 2000-2006. In 2002, he was awarded the Canadian Liver Foundation Commemorative Medal for the Queen's Jubilee for his contribution to liver disease in Canada. In 2005, he was the recipient of the Ivan T. Beck Research Lectureship for his outstanding contribution to research in gastroenterology and hepatology nationally and internationally. From 2004 to 2007 he served on the International Committee of the American Gastroenterology Association. In 2006 he received the Graduate Course Director Award from the Institute of Medical Science at the University of Toronto and was appointed to the Board of the Stem Cell Network. He recently joined the University of Toronto Medical Journal Faculty Advisory Board for 2007-08.

In July 2008 he was appointed as the first Director of the newly formed University of Toronto Transplant Institute.

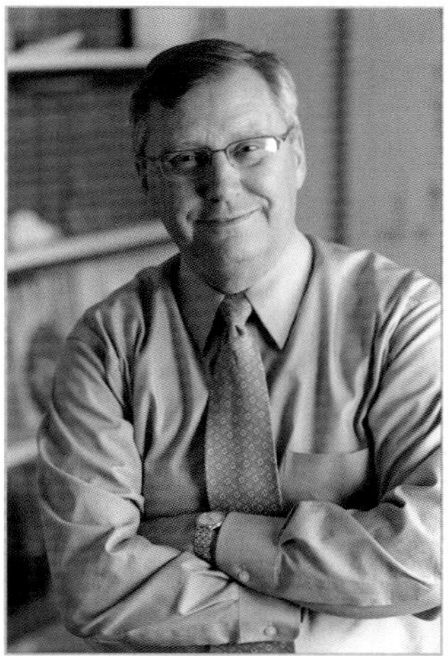

John R. Lake, MD

University of Minnesota Medical Center
Fairview, Minnesota USA

John R. Lake, MD, is the Director of the Liver Transplantation Program and Executive Medical Director of the Solid Organ Transplantation Program at the University of Minnesota Medical Center. He is an internationally known transplant hepatologist and active member of nine medical societies.

In 1999, Dr. Lake was the first transplant hepatologist to serve as president of the American Society of Transplantation, and he currently serves on the board of the United Network for Organ Sharing (UNOS) and the council of the International Liver Transplantation Society.

Dr. Lake has published extensively, with over 170 scientific papers, 20 reviews and 25 book chapters to his credit. His research interests include post-transplant hepatitis C and outcome predictors for liver transplant results. He also works to develop new immunosuppressive agents.

Dr. Lake is a Deputy Editor for the *American Journal of Transplantation* and will become the editor of *Liver Transplantation* in July. He has served as an *ad hoc* reviewer, guest editor, editorial board member and/or associate editor for nearly 20 publications. He has also volunteered on 25 community or national committees related to transplantation.

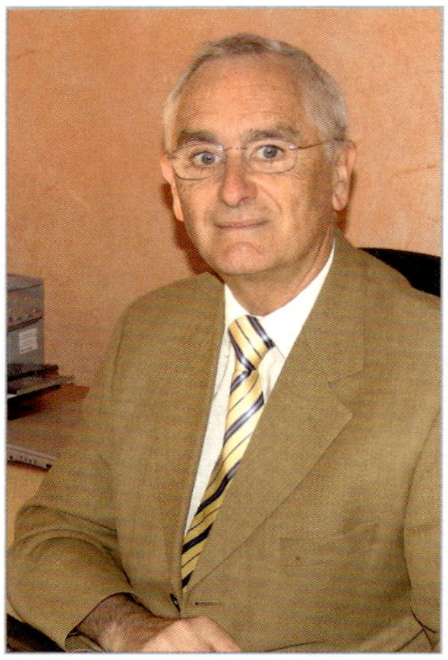

David W. Holt, DSc (Med), FRCPath

St. George's, University of London, UK

David Holt is the Director of the Analytical Unit and Professor of Bioanalytics at St George's, University of London, UK. He has more than 38 years' experience in the measurement of drugs as a guide to therapy, and has been responsible for the development of assays used to monitor a wide variety of therapeutic agents. Following a doctoral thesis on the measurement of digoxin he has been involved in definitive clinical pharmacokinetic studies of antiarrhythmic drugs, in particular amiodarone, and a broad range of immunosuppressive drugs. Currently, he is involved in the measurement of endogenous compounds associated with cardiovascular diseases as biomarkers of disease progression, and in the rapidly expanding field of pharmacogenetics. He is also responsible for Forensic Toxicology Services at St George's, where he provides services to HM Coroners, pathologists and law enforcement agencies for the analysis of illicit and prescription drugs.

Professor Holt has advised on several consensus panels on immunosuppressive drug monitoring and is widely known as the organiser of International Proficiency Testing Schemes for immunosuppressive drugs. He is a member of the Steering Committee of the UK National External Quality Assessment Schemes (NEQAS) for Drug Measurements. His current research interests include the development of mass-spectrometric assays for the measurement of endogenous markers of organ damage and dysfunction, pharmacogenetics, the development of methods to assess phenotypic markers of drug metabolism and the detection of drugs used in drug-facilitated crime. He is a frequent speaker on a broad range of issues relating to bioanalytics and clinical toxicology, and is the author of over 300 publications in peer reviewed journals and invited contributions to books. He is an active member of several national and international scientific societies involved in transplantation and cardiology and he is The Past President of the International Association of Therapeutic Drug Monitoring and Clinical Toxicology.

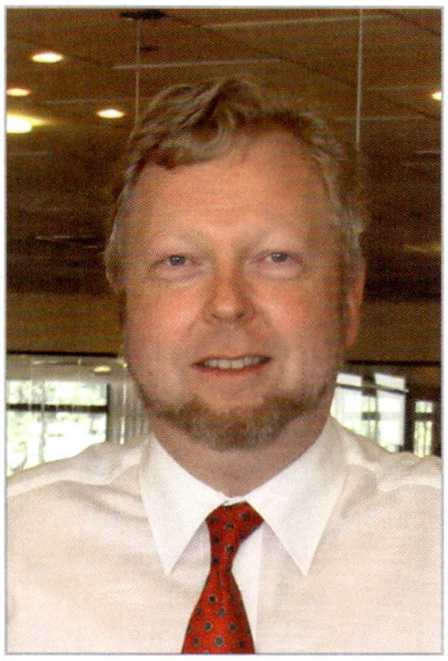

Pierre Wallemacq, PhD, EurClin Chem

Cliniques Universitaires St Luc, UCL,
Brussels, Belgium

Dr. Pierre Wallemacq, PhD is Professor at the Université Catholique de Louvain, Medical School in Brussels, Belgium. He teaches clinical chemistry, toxicology and clinical pharmacokinetics, and is the vice president of the biomedical sciences school. He is responsible for a research unit (LBCM) in the Medical School and supervises several PhD theses and post-doc fellows. He is also head of laboratory in the Cliniques Universitaires St Luc, Brussels, in charge of the analytical biochemistry platform regrouping activities such as TDM, clinical toxicology, forensic toxicology, but also special chemistry (GC, HPLC, UPLC, LC-MSMS, GC-MS). He started working in the field of TDM in 1982 with his PhD thesis on cyclosporine, and is author or co-author of more than 130 peer-reviewed manuscripts and nine textbook chapters. He has presented at more than 170 conferences on invitation and has been an invited professor at several universities including the Pontifícia Universidade Católica do Rio Grande do Sul or PUCRS (Porto Alegre) and the Centro Universitario Feevale (Novo Hamburgo), in Brazil. Most of his work was dedicated to immunosuppressive drugs, and he also published works in other clinical chemistry TDM/TOX areas. Pierre Wallemacq was elected President of the Royal Belgian Society of Clinical Chemistry (SBCC-BVKC) in 2008, and President of the Belgian and Luxemburg Society of Toxicology (BLT) in 2007. He is a member of the editorial boards of several international journals such as *Therapeutic Drug Monitoring* (TDM), *Clinical Biochemistry* (CLB), *Clinical Chemistry and Laboratory Medicine* (CCLM). Effective July 2009 he will be an associate editor for *Clinical Biochemistry*. He has served as a guest editor, and has been involved as a member of the scientific organization committees of several international congresses. Recently, he was elected Director of Education in the International Association of Therapeutic Drug Monitoring and Clinical Toxicology (IATDMCT).

A

Acute rejection

Immunologic graft rejection which occurs early, usually within the first year of transplantation, and is generally reversible with additional immunosuppressive medication.

Alkaline Phosphatase (ALP)

An enzyme released into the blood of patients with liver or bone disease.

Alloimmune response

Immunologic reaction of the immune system against the allograft.

Anemia

Low red blood cell count.

Antibody dependent toxicity

Production of antibodies which bind to cells and cause their destruction, for example, antibodies produced against the donor graft by the allograft recipient.

Apoptosis

Programmed controlled cell death.

Area Under the Time-Concentration Curve (AUC)

Measurement of the concentration of a drug in whole blood or plasma after intake integrated over time post-dosing. The area under this curve is considered the best marker of drug exposure.

Ascites

Accumulation of fluid in the peritoneal cavity commonly due to cirrhosis and liver disease.

Aspartate Transaminase (AST)

An enzyme released into the blood during heptocellular necrosis, i.e. liver damage.

Assay sensitivity

A term used to define the smallest amount of an analyte that can be reliably measured by an assay.

Assay specificity

The ability of an assay to detect the analyte of interest and not detect analytes with a similar chemical structure or analytes that interfere in the signal detection process. Common problems relate to distinguishing between the parent drug and drug metabolites.

Atherosclerosis

Progressive disease characterized by thickening of the arterial wall due to the deposition of fatty materials.

B

Basophils

The least abundant white blood cell that stains dark blue with hematoxylin and eosin (H&E) dyes capable of ingesting foreign material and is associated with asthma and allergies. Part of the polymorphonuclear cell family (PMN), together with eosinophils and neutrophils.

Biopsy Proven Acute Rejection (BPAR)

Removal and examination of allograft tissue which demonstrates the presence of immune cells invading the donor organ.

Bland-Altman plot

A scatter plot used to assess the agreement between two clinical methods by plotting the difference between methods against their mean values.

C

C_0

Measurement of the trough concentration of a drug in whole blood or plasma, usually the lowest concentration before the next dose.

C_2

Measurement of the concentration of a drug in whole blood or plasma 2 hours after intake.

C4d

A component of the complement cascade and degradation product of C4.

Cardiovascular disease

A spectrum of diseases of the heart and vasculature including narrowing of the blood vessels of the heart (arteriosclerosis).

Calcineurin

Protein phosphatase inhibited by a complex of immunophilin and cyclosporine or tacrolimus, responsible for dephosphorylation of NFAT, a transcription factor regulating the production of IL-2.

Choledocho-choledochstomy

Method of biliary reconstruction following orthotopic liver transplantation.

Chronic Allograft Nephropathy (CAN)

Progressive tissue damage to the kidney resulting in gradual renal failure due to immune and non-immune factors.

Chronic Obstructive Pulmonary Disease (COPD)

Lung diseases that block airflow and make it difficult to breathe, e.g. emphysema, chronic bronchitis.

Chronic rejection

Immunologic graft rejection which occurs later, generally after the first year of transplantation, is not reversible and leads to progressive loss of allograft function.

Chronic renal failure

Progressive and irreversible loss of renal function.

Complement

A collection of proteins capable of lysing microorganisms, infected cells, and cells recognized as foreign by the immune system.

Corticosteroids

Anti-inflammatory drugs used to suppress the immune system.

Critical Dose Drug

A drug for which small changes in dose can result in changes in drug exposure, leading either to toxicity or loss of efficacy.

Cytochrome P450

Major family of enzymes which are responsible for drug metabolism. These enzymes oxidize drugs to make them more water soluble so they can be excreted into the bile or urine.

Cytokines

A class of secreted, signaling proteins which regulate the immune response, inflammation, and hematopoiesis.

Cytotoxic T cell response

The induction of apoptosis by T cells which recognize the display of foreign antigens by MHC on the surface of a cell.

D

Delayed graft function

Insufficient renal function following transplantation requiring dialysis.

Delayed type hypersensitivity

A process which can take 1-3 days caused by antigen-sensitized effector T cells when they encounter their specific antigen and begin recruitment of macrophages.

Deming regression

A method of linear regression which accounts for error in measurements in both x and y variables.

Diabetes mellitus

Metabolic disorder characterized by hyperglycemia due to lack of insulin or insulin resistance.

Ductopenia

Reduction in the number of bile ducts.

E

Endovascular ultrasonography

The use of ultrasound to probe the vasculature.

Eosinophils

White blood cells that stain brick-red with eosin dye, responsible for combating infection. Part of the polymorphonuclear cell family (PMN), together with basophils and neutrophils.

F

FLOW cytometry (FACS)

A method for sorting and counting cells in an aqueous fluid stream. Fluorescence Activated Cell Sorting uses the light scattering and fluorescence properties of cells to sort them into different containers.

G

Glomerular Filtration Rate (GFR)

A measure of renal function usually calculated from serum creatinine concentration.

H

Hemolytic-uremic syndrome

A triad of diseases which include hemolytic anemia, acute renal failure, and thrombocytopenia.

Hemophilia

Bleeding disorder characterized by the inability of the blood to clot properly.

Hepatic encephalopathy

Disease of the brain caused by severe liver impairment.

Hepatic or Intestinal First-Pass Effect

Metabolism of a drug by the Cytochrome P450 enzymes present in hepatocytes or enterocytes, thereby reducing the amount of the parent drug which reaches the systemic circulation.

Hepatitis

Inflammation of the liver.

Hepatitis C Virus (HCV)

A lipoprotein-enveloped RNA virus which belongs to the Flaviviridae family and is a major cause of chronic hepatitis, liver cirrhosis and hepatocellular carcinoma. End-stage liver disease caused by HCV is the main indication for liver transplantation.

Hepatocellular carcinoma

Cancer of the liver.

Hepatosplenomegaly

Simultaneous enlargement of both the liver and spleen.

Human Immunodeficiency Virus (HIV)

A lentivirus which belongs to the retrovirus family which causes acquired immunodeficiency syndrome (AIDS). HIV destroys cellular immunity by the depletion of CD4+ T cells which results in the progressive loss of immunity and protection from infectious diseases.

Humoral immune response

Production of antibody by B cells against specific antigens.

Human Leukocyte Antigen (HLA)

Proteins which display peptides derived from inside the cell onto the outside surface of the cell. HLA is the human species version of the Major Histocompatibility Complex (MHC) found in vertebrates.

Hyperlipidemia

Elevated lipids and lipoproteins in the blood.

Hypertension

Elevated blood pressure.

I

Immunophilins

Cytoplasmic proteins which bind cyclosporine or tacrolimus resulting in blocking the phosphatase activity of calcineurin.

Immunosuppression

Prevention or interference with the development of the normal immunologic response which can occur through disease causing agents and various drugs and chemicals.

Induction therapy

The use of potent immunosuppressive antibodies given intravenously at the time of transplantation to rapidly achieve a state of immunosuppression.

Innate immune response

A non-specific, antigen-independent defense mechanism to infection which is always present and readily mobilized during infection.

Interleukin 2 (IL-2)

Cytokine produced during an immune response which triggers the proliferation of T cells.

Ischemia-reperfusion injury

Restriction of the blood supply (ischemia) to an organ removed from a donor causes tissue damage. Upon transplantation of the organ and return of the blood supply, white blood cells release pro-inflammatory cytokines in response to this damage causing further damage.

J

Jaundice

Yellowish discoloration of the skin due to hyperbilirubinemia.

L

Leukopenia

Low white blood cell count.

Limit of Detection (LOD)

The lowest concentration of an analyte that can be distinguished from background.

Liver cirrhosis

Progressive deterioration of the liver due to chronic injury. Development of scar tissue impairs the ability of the liver to function.

Lower Limit of Quantification (LLOQ)

The lowest concentration of an analyte that can be reliably measured, usually defined as the concentration at which the coefficient of variance (CV) of the concentration measured is no more than 20%. For chromatographic assays the LLOQ is usually the concentration of the lowest calibrator.

Lymphocytes

A class of white blood cells composed of B cells (humoral immunity), T cells and NK cells (cellular immunity).

M

Macrophages

White blood cells derived from monocytes which engulf foreign material and are also involved in antigenic stimulation.

Maintenance therapy

The use of orally administered immunosuppressive drugs after transplantation to maintain adequate immunosuppression and prevent rejection. These drugs are usually taken throughout the life of an allograft recipient.

Mammalian Target of Rapamycin (mTOR)

A serine/threonine protein kinase which regulates cell growth and is inhibited by the binding of the immunosuppressive drugs sirolimus (rapamycin) and everolimus.

Metabolic bone disease

General term for a variety of disorders that cause bone abnormalities.

Mitogen Activated Protein Kinase pathway (MAPK)

A complex pathway composed of many proteins and protein kinases responsible for signal transduction coupling of growth factors binding to cell surface receptors with intracellular activities, e.g. gene transcription.

Monocytes

White blood cells which differentiate into macrophages and dendritic cells to fight infection.

N

Neoplasia

The abnormal uncontrolled proliferation of cells.

Nephrotoxic

Chemicals or drugs poisonous to kidney cells.

Neurotoxic

Chemicals or drugs poisonous to cells of the nervous system.

Neutropenia

Abnormally low number of neutrophil granulocytes which make up 50-70% of the white cell count. Neutrophils destroy bacteria in the blood.

Neutrophil Gelatinase-Associated Lipocalin (NGAL)

This is a protein produced by neutrophils that is elevated in the serum of patients with bacterial infection, asthma, or Chronic Obstructive Pulmonary Disease (COPD). Elevated concentrations of NGAL in blood and urine have been observed in patients with renal disease.

Neutrophils

The most abundant white blood cell that stains neutral pink with hematoxylin and eosin (H&E) dyes, responsible for phagocytosis of microorganisms or particles. Part of the polymorphonuclear cell family (PMN), together with eosinophils and basophils.

NK cells

Natural Killer cytotoxic lymphocytes that can induce cell apoptosis or necrosis without specific antigen recognition. These cells are part of the innate immune system.

O

Once daily (od, qd)

Drug dose administered one time per day.

Oral bioavailability

Fraction of the parent drug that reaches the systemic circulation after oral intake.

Orthotopic liver transplantation (OLT)

Replacement of a diseased liver with a healthy donor liver in the same location.

Osteoporosis

Disease characterized by progressive bone loss leading to increased risk of bone fracture.

P

Passing-Bablok regression

A method of linear regression which accounts for error in measurements in both x and y variables, does not assume the error is normally distributed, and is robust against outlier data points.

Pharmacodynamics

Studies the effect the drug has on the body.

Pharmacogenetics

Studies the differences in gene structure (nucleotide polymorphisms) with pharmacologic differences in drug metabolism, transport, or pharmacodynamic action.

Pharmacokinetics

Studies the effect the body has on the drug.

Plasmapheresis

Method used to separate blood plasma from blood cells.

Platelets

Anuclear cells responsible for blood clot formation.

Polyoma Virus (BK virus)

A nonenveloped DNA virus which belongs to the polyomavirus family and is a serious cause of nephropathy in some renal allograft recipients.

Protein kinase C (PKC)

A family of phospholipid-dependent serine/threonine protein kinases that are involved in signal transduction activities associated with cell differentiation, proliferation, and apoptosis.

Proteinuria

Protein in urine.

Prothrombin Time and International Normalization Ratio (PT/INR)

Test used to evaluate the ability of the blood to clot properly. The INR is used to monitor the effect of anti-coagulant drugs, i.e. to ensure adequate clot prevention without excessive bleeding.

Pneumonitis

Inflammation of the lung tissue.

S

Scleral icterus

Yellowish discoloration of the sclerae (whites of the eyes) due to hyperbilirubinemia.

Sclerotherapy

Procedure to treat blood vessel abnormalities or malformations. This procedure can be used to treat variceal bleeding.

Serum creatinine

Surrogate marker for GFR (renal function).

Serum cryoglobulins

Immunoglobulins in serum that undergo reversible precipitation at low temperatures, that can be associated with chronic viral hepatitis.

Single Nucleotide Polymorphisms (SNPs)

The variation of a single nucleotide in a gene or DNA sequence between members of the same species.

T

Therapeutic Drug Monitoring (TDM)

Repeated measurement of the concentration of a drug in whole blood or plasma as a guide to drug dosing.

Thrombocytopenia

Low platelet count.

Thymocyte

Cells which develop in the thymus and are precursors to mature T cells.

Twice daily (bid)

Drug dose administered two times per day.

V

Variceal bleeding

Increased pressure in the portal vein caused by blockage in the flow of blood through the liver results in the development of large veins to bypass the blocked area. These large veins (varices) are fragile and are prone to bleed.

Viral cardiomyopathy

Viral persistence in the heart which can lead to cardiac damage.

W

White Blood Cells (WBC)

Cells in the blood which fight infection and include basophils, eosinophils, lymphocytes (B and T cells), monocytes, and neutrophils.